CW00970396

Successful Periodontal Therapy
A Non-Surgical Approach

Quintessentials of Dental Practice – 16
Periodontology - 3

Successful Periodontal Therapy

A Non-Surgical Approach

By
Peter A Heasman
Philip M Preshaw
Pauline Robertson

Editor-in-Chief: Nairn H F Wilson
Editor Periodontology: Iain L C Chapple

Quintessence Publishing Co. Ltd.

London, Berlin, Chicago, Copenhagen, Paris, Milan, Barcelona,
Istanbul, São Paulo, Tokyo, New Dehli, Moscow, Prague, Warsaw

British Library Cataloguing in Publication Data

Heasman, Peter A.
    Successful periodontal therapy : a non-surgical approach. -
    (Quintessentials of dental practice. Periodontology ; 16. Periodontology ; 3)
    1. Periodontal disease - Treatment
    I.Title II.Preshaw, Philip III.Robertson, Pauline
    617.6'3206

    ISBN 1850970742

Copyright © 2004 Quintessence Publishing Co. Ltd., London

Figs 4-1, 4-3, 4-5 by Laura Andrew

All rights reserved. This book or any part thereof may not be reproduced,
stored in a retrieval system, or transmitted in any form or by any
means, electronic, mechanical, photocopying, or otherwise, without the written
permission of the publisher.

ISBN 1-85097-074-2

Foreword

Successful periodontal therapy is, for many, fundamental to the goal of teeth for life. With a state-of-the-art non-surgical approach to periodontal therapy, success is dependent on a plethora of interrelated factors and influences, including the complexity of the disease process, predisposing risk factors, diagnostic skills and techniques, patient management and motivation, knowledge of modern instrumentation, techniques and adjunctive treatments, not to forget clinical acumen both during active treatment and the equally critical long-term supportive periodontal care. Can all of this be covered effectively in a slim, easy-to-read book? Yes, it can: the authors of Volume 16, Periodontology 3 in the Quintessentials of Dental Practice Series have achieved this feat, with plenty extra packed in by way of a bonus.

It is proving to be a great learning experience being Editor-in-Chief of the Quintessentials of Dental Practice Series, the present book having added greatly to my new enlightenment. Dental students, trainee hygienists and therapists and practitioners of all ages, not to forget everyone's patients, will benefit enormously from this timely contribution to the existing literature. I hope you enjoy and learn from this excellent book as much as I did.

Nairn Wilson
Editor-in-Chief

Preface

This text is the third of five books that aim to provide the general dental practitioner with an illustrated practical and contemporary guide to the management of patients with gingival and periodontal diseases. This book is entitled *Successful Periodontal Therapy: A Non-Surgical Approach*. Initially it presents the reader with recognised goals and objectives of non-surgical treatment. Subsequent chapters cover the clinical protocols and methods for achieving these goals: hygiene phase; scaling and root surface instrumentation; the instruments used for scaling and root surface debridement; managing common and well-established risk-factors; and the use of treatments that are considered to be adjunctive to conventional methods of scaling and root surface instrumentation. The final chapter reviews the importance of supportive periodontal care, which is highly relevant for general dental practitioners, for both those patients that they have treated in the primary care setting and those who may have received their non-surgical management by a specialist or in a hospital environment.

The Aim

It is hoped that having read this book on periodontal therapy the reader will be able to:
- understand the healing events that follow non-surgical treatment
- realise the limitations of non-surgical treatment
- have knowledge of the range of mechanical and chemical products that are available to improve personal plaque control
- be aware of the range of instruments that are available for removing tooth deposits
- understand the importance of identifying and managing systemic and local risk factors for periodontal diseases
- understand the importance of identifying and managing local anatomical and iatrogenic factors that may predispose to periodontal disease
- be aware of systemic and locally-delivered adjunctive treatments that are available and know how to reach informed decisions regarding the most appropriate product for any specific clinical situation
- understand the goals of supportive periodontal care and how they might be achieved

- appreciate the need for patient compliance and understand how poor patient compliance might be identified and improved.

Peter Heasman
Philip Preshaw
Pauline Robertson
Iain Chapple

Acknowledgements

The authors would like to acknowledge with sincere thanks the following people: Janet Howarth of the Department of Dental Photography at Newcastle Dental Hospital for her photographic expertise; Dr David Jacobs for Fig 5-1; Dr Shakil Shahdad for Figs 5-2 and 5-3; Dr Robert Wassell for Fig 5-5; Dr Dean Barker for Figs 5-8, 5-9 and 5-10; Dentsply UK for Figs 3-4, 3-6, 3-7, 3-9, 3-10 and 3-14. We are grateful also to Professor Iain Chapple for Figs 3-15, 5-7 and 5-11 and Mrs Suzanne Noble for use of Figs 3-16, 3-17 and 3-18. Permission has been granted to reproduce the following: Fig 2-4 (from Heasman, Millett, Chapple. *The Periodontium and Orthodontics in Health and Disease*. Oxford; Oxford University Press: 1996); Fig 5-5 (from Barnes, Walls. *Gerodontology*. Oxford; Wright: 1994); Fig 5-20 (from Heasman, Preshaw, Smith. *Periodontology Colour Guide*. London; Churchill Livingstone: 1997). Thanks to Iain Chapple and Damien Walmsley for the cover photograph and to George Warman Publications, publishers of *Dental Update*, for permission to reprint part of this image.

Professor Heasman would like to acknowledge the support of Lynne, Sophie and Christopher, during the preparation of this book. Dr Preshaw would like to thank his wife, Sarah, for her help and support. Pauline Robertson would like to acknowledge the support of her husband, Brian, and family.

Contents

Chapter 1
The Goals and Clinical Outcomes of Non-Surgical Treatment

Aims

This chapter aims to outline the goals of non-surgical periodontal treatment and to provide an overview of the clinical outcomes that are expected following treatment.

Outcome

After reading this chapter the practitioner should have an understanding of:
- the healing events that follow non-surgical treatment
- the magnitude of the clinical changes and outcomes expected following the hygiene (or initial) and instrumentation (or corrective) phases
- the limitations of non-surgical treatment.

The Periodontal Pocket – A Pathological Environment

A periodontal pocket is a pathologically deepened gingival crevice. The lateral and apical boundaries of the pocket are the ulcerated epithelial lining of the pocket wall and the junctional epithelium respectively. The remaining "wall" of the defect comprises the diseased root surface – the "target" for periodontal treatment.

The diseased root surface is contaminated with subgingival calculus deposits and a layer of dental plaque, which contains the periodontal pathogens that constantly challenge and compromise the host's defence mechanisms. Dental plaque is now regarded as a biofilm, which essentially is an organised community of bacteria that forms on a non-shedding surface such as a tooth. Bacteria attach to the tooth and produce a matrix of extracellular polymers to help bind them together. Microcolonies form and new species join the biofilm which then contains diverse species and metabolic states. Gingival crevicular fluid (GCF) flows through the many channels in the aggregation to provide nutrients and to remove some of the waste products. The biofilm is viable and bacteria can proliferate to establish new colonies on other parts of the root surface.

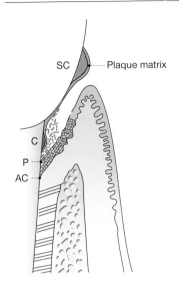

Fig 1-1 Diagrammatic representation of a periodontal pocket for a patient with chronic periodontitis. The pocket epithelium, which is ulcerated, has migrated down on to the root surface. Calculus deposits are present both supra- and subgingivally and these deposits are covered with a layer of plaque. The subgingival plaque may also be regarded as a biofilm with a complex population of loosely adherent micro-organisms on its surface.

SC, supragingival calculus

C, subgingival calculus

P, the most apical extent of the periodontal pocket

AC, the most apical cell of the junctional epithelium

The majority of bacteria in an established biofilm are recognised, anaerobic organisms with cell walls containing powerful lipopolysaccharide (LPS) based endotoxins. Studies have shown that the vast majority of LPS is only loosely bound to, or associated with, the root surfaces although a small percentage of the total LPS may cause subsurface contamination, in particular at sites of root surface irregularities, root grooves or resorption lacunae. Subgingival calculus on the root surface may also be contaminated with LPS. Diagrammatic representations of a diseased root surface are shown in Fig 1-1.

The Aims of Non-Surgical Treatment

The overall aim of non-surgical treatment is to create an environment that is biologically compatible with healing of the periodontal tissues. This is most likely to be achieved by:

- decontamination by removing LPS/endotoxins from the root surface
- disrupting and eliminating the biofilm from the root surface
- removing the bulk of subgingival calculus from the root surface.

Laboratory studies have shown that a gentle stream of water can remove about 39% of the LPS whilst brushing the root surface eliminates a further 60%. This suggests that the hygiene phase of non-surgical treatment may be instrumental in disrupting the biofilm and eliminating up to 99% of endo-

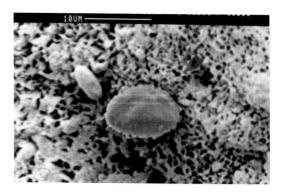

Fig 1-2 Scanning electron microscope view of a periodontally involved root surface showing porous and necrotic cementum.

toxins in the pocket. Such a hypothesis of course makes the assumption that the patient is able to access the entire depth of the pocket during cleaning. This is seldom achieved for pockets that are greater than 5mm in depth. Indeed, the deeper the pocket, the more residual, undisturbed biofilm is likely to remain.

The need for professional intervention is, therefore, crucial and this includes root surface instrumentation, a term which is used in preference to root planing. Root surface instrumentation describes the procedure that is necessary to eliminate endotoxins, disrupt the biofilm and, when present, remove subgingival calculus from the root surface (also called root surface debridement). Root surfaces that have no detectable subgingival calculus may be instrumented by passing an instrument such as an ultrasonic scaler lightly over the surface. This will remove the loosely associated toxins and the majority of the outermost, necrotic cementum on the root surface (Fig 1-2). Research shows that the most effective use of ultrasonic instruments involves multiple light passes of the instrument over the root surface. The presence of tenacious, subgingival calculus will, however, necessitate the use of greater pressure to the root, although the belief that the root surface has to be meticulously "planed" until it is hard and smooth is now largely outdated.

Elimination of Calculus

Calculus is not the cause of periodontal disease, but may be regarded as a contributory factor, for several reasons including:
- all calculus has a coating layer of dental plaque
- supragingival calculus impedes toothbrushing and interdental cleaning

3

- subgingival calculus may act as both a barrier to subgingival cleaning and a focus for the colonization of bacteria during the first stage in the formation of a biofilm
- subgingival calculus may absorb bacterial endotoxins
- supra- and subgingival calculus may impede the passage of periodontal probes, thereby falsifying borderline probing depth measures.

For these reasons, it is important to try to remove as much of the calculus as possible, although some residual, isolated deposits of subgingival calculus are likely to be compatible with periodontal healing. This observation is consistent with studies that have shown that even under optimal conditions of access during periodontal surgery absolutely calculus-free root surfaces following root surface instrumentation are hardly ever achieved. With the understanding that pockets with probing depths of >5mm are exceptionally difficult to render plaque and calculus free, it is almost certain that residual deposits are more likely to be the rule rather than the exception with a non-surgical approach.

The Concept of Full-Mouth Disinfection

The importance of eliminating the biofilm and bacteria that have freedom of movement around the oral cavity, and are the cause of periodontal infections and re-infections, has been recognised by the introduction of full-mouth disinfection as a novel treatment strategy for periodontal diseases. Full-mouth disinfection involves the conventional removal of root surface deposits, usually over two visits within 24 hours of one another. Instruction in oral hygiene procedures is also given at one or both visits. This treatment recognises, however, that many of the potent pathogens, such as *Porphyromonas gingivalis* and *Actinobacillus actinomycetemcomitans,* are also commonly found at non-periodontal sites such as on the dorsum of the tongue, on the oral mucosa, in saliva, or on the mucosal surface of the tonsils. Re-infection of treated pockets is, therefore, likely unless an attempt is made to eliminate the organisms from all of these niches and as quickly as possible. The fewer the number of visits, the less chance there is for re-infection from (as yet) untreated sites.

Different preparations of chlorhexidine gluconate have also been used in an attempt to achieve adjunctive disinfection immediately after the completion of root surface instrumentation (Table 1-1). There is little evidence, however, to support the clinical value of the adjunctive use of chlorhexidine over mechanical instrumentation alone during full-mouth disinfection.

Table 1-1 **Preparations of chlorhexidine gluconate that have been used to help achieve full-mouth disinfection after root surface instrumentation.**

Preparation	Application
1% gel	Brushing the dorsum of the tongue for 1 minute
0.2% mouth rinse	Full-mouth rinse for 1 minute
0.2% spray	Applied to the tonsil region
1% gel	Repeated (x 3) subgingival irrigation over a 10-minute period
0.2% mouth rinse	Twice-daily rinse for 1 minute at home for 2 months
0.2% spray	Twice-daily application to tonsil region for 2 months

Healing Following Periodontal Treatment

One of the principal signs of a healing pocket is the reduction in probing depth that follows treatment. This reduction is largely a result of the resolution of gingival inflammation leading to shrinkage of the gingival tissues and the formation of a new, long junctional epithelium (Fig 1-3).

Supragingival scaling, prophylaxis and the removal of dental plaque as a consequence of improved plaque control by the patient reduce the bacterial challenge to the host and, as a result, there is a resolution of the acute inflammatory lesion in the gingival tissues. These changes may occur within 1-2 weeks and are characterised by reductions in gingival swelling, redness and gingival bleeding (Fig 1-4).

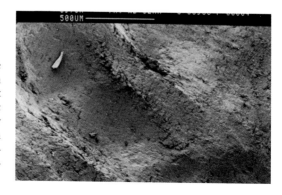

Fig 1-3 The root surface shown in Fig 1-2 has been instrumented using light application of an ultrasonic scaler. The root surface is now relatively smooth, although there are noticeable indentations as a result of the instrumentation.

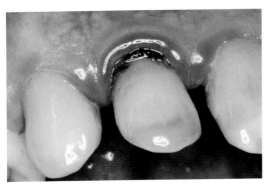

Fig 1-4 A band of calculus on the labial aspect of a maxillary incisor. This calculus has the typical appearance of a sub-gingival deposit. This deposit has now become supragingival due to resolution of gingival inflammation following hygiene-phase therapy. Note that the free gingival margin is still inflamed because the calculus has a surface layer of dental plaque.

Efficient root surface instrumentation and disruption of the subgingival biofilm will create a root surface that is biologically compatible with the formation of the long junctional epithelium. The new epithelium adheres to the root surface through a hemidesmosomal attachment between the cells and the surface cementum. These epithelial cells are derived from the remaining apical healthy junctional epithelium and some of the pocket epithelium that retains the potential for regeneration. This contributes to the healing process once the bacterial challenge to the host is removed. The attachment of epithelium begins within a few days of root surface instrumentation at the most apical extremity of the pocket and then progresses coronally over 2-3 weeks. Maturation of the gingival and periodontal collagen fibres then follows. Although there is no new connective tissue attachment of principal periodontal fibres to the root surface, these later changes enhance the integrity of the tissues to further reduce the probing depths.

The reduction of gingival swelling and enlargement leads to supragingival exposure of root surfaces that have to be maintained as part of the supportive periodontal care programme: regular prophylaxis, application of fluoride varnish and, if necessary, desensitising agents (Chapter 7). The post-treatment morphology of the gingival tissue is often irregular and may further complicate plaque control and provide another challenge to patients who are already adept at interproximal and subgingival cleaning (Fig 1-8).

Clinical Outcomes Following Non-Surgical Treatment

It is now accepted that non-surgical treatment for a motivated and compliant patient is likely to result in some improvement in periodontal status irrespective of the severity of chronic periodontitis and the probing depths at

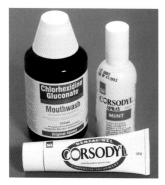

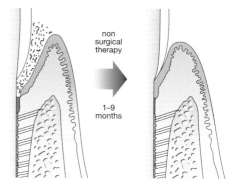

Fig 1-5 Preparations of chlorhexidine gluconate used for full mouth disinfection: mouthwash, spray and gel.

Fig 1-6 Diagrammatic representation outlining the healing mechanisms after non-surgical therapy. Following removal of the aetiological dental plaque, there has been resolution of gingival inflammation (and gingival shrinkage), and hemi-desmosomal attachment of epithelial cells to the biologically compatible root surface. This healing process may take up to nine months to complete.

diagnosis. It was only during the 1980s that data were reported in a series of classical, longitudinal clinical trials, to document for the first time the changes that might be expected following both the hygiene and instrumentation stages of non-surgical management (Fig 1-6).

Hygiene versus instrumentation phases

The study by Cercek and his colleagues at Loma Linda University in 1983, reported the relative effects of plaque control and root surface instrumentation on patients with chronic periodontitis (Fig 1-7). The *hygiene phase* comprised twice-daily toothbrushing and the use of floss and interdental brushes where appropriate. The clinical effects were:

- significant reductions in plaque score within one month of treatment. Initial scores of 60% at shallow pockets were reduced to 5% whereas the deeper pockets with plaque scores of around 90% showed reductions of 10-15%
- a reduction of BoP from 70% to 40% within three months
- an average reduction of probing depth of approximately 0.5mm
- some loss of clinical attachment.

The bleeding scores were reduced to a greater extent in shallow pockets (≤3.5mm) than in deeper pockets (≥6mm) because of the limited access of

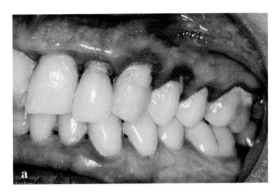

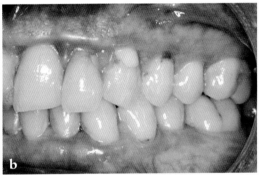

Fig 1-7a Gingival inflammation is present in a patient with chronic periodontitis;
b The same patient two weeks later following instruction in toothbrushing. Supragingival calculus has also been removed but, at this stage, methods for interdental cleaning have not been introduced. Some supragingival plaque deposits remain, although the level of plaque control has improved considerably and, as a result, the aggressive nature of the gingival inflammation has resolved.

brushes and floss to those deeper sites. The deeper sites did, however, demonstrate greater reductions in probing depths than the shallow sites. Deeper sites tend to have more acute inflammation and swelling of the gingiva when compared to the shallower sites and, therefore, have more potential for gingival recession following improvements in plaque control. A slight loss of attachment (about 0.1mm) tended to occur at the deeper sites because of the lack of effectiveness of plaque control measures at the base of pockets. Loss of attachment at the shallower sites occurred because of local trauma from improved tooth cleaning measures that are able to access the depth of the pockets.

Further changes followed the *instrumentation phase* that comprised one episode of root surface instrumentation using an ultrasonic scaler. These observations were:

- continued reductions in probing depths of up to 1mm with the initially deeper pockets showing greater reductions than the shallower pockets

Fig 1-8 An irregular gingival morphology at interproximal sites between maxillary incisors and canine. The gingival shrinkage that has occurred will make it easier for the patient to use interdental aids to maintain a high level of plaque control, even though the gingival morphology is irregular.

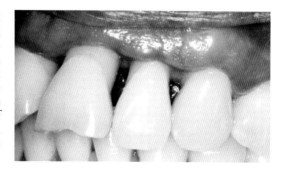

Fig 1-9 Graph showing expected resolution of bleeding on probing and probing depths following non-surgical treatment in patients with advanced chronic periodontitis. Percentage of bleeding sites falls from 100 to approximately 20% during the first six months following treatment. Mean probing depths may have reduced from 8mm to approximately 5mm. Note that a 5mm pocket that does

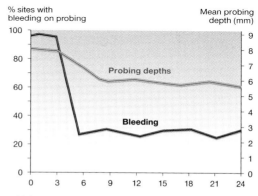

not bleed following probing should be maintained through a programme of supportive periodontal care. Pockets that continue to bleed following treatment should be inspected carefully for residual calculus and plaque deposits and, if present, retreatment will be indicated (after Badersten, Nilveus, Egelberg 1984).

- improved attachment levels for the initially deep pockets but not for the shallower pockets (<3mm prior to treatment), which are susceptible to loss of attachment following both the hygiene and instrumentation phases.

These data show clearly that clinical improvement does occur following the hygiene phase of treatment, but the changes are likely to be limited, in particular in pockets of 4mm or greater. If the clinical changes are to be maximised then root surface instrumentation is essential.

The Badersten studies
In the 1980s, Anita Badersten and her colleagues, at Loma Linda University, reported a series of clinical trials that studied the healing events and clin-

ical outcomes following non-surgical treatment in patients with moderate and advanced chronic periodontitis. These studies did not allow a detailed, separate interpretation of the effects of the hygiene and instrumentation phases and only incisors, canines and premolars were included in the studies. Nevertheless, despite these limitations, the studies provided the first, indepth report of clinical outcomes following non-surgical treatment of moderate and advanced chronic periodontitis (Figs 1-7 to 1-9). The principal outcomes and conclusions are shown in Table 1-2.

An evidence base for non-surgical treatment

Hung and Douglass published a meta-analysis of the effects of root surface instrumentation. This type of analysis allows the results from several studies to be combined so that overall trends of clinical outcomes can be identified. Nine studies were included in the analysis because specified inclusion criteria were set after the research was carried out and, as with any review of this nature, many studies were excluded. For example, one inclusion criterion was that probing depths had to be stratified into shallow (1-3mm), moderate (4-6mm) or deep (>7mm) at the outset.

The summary points from the analysis were consistent with the findings of the Cercek and Badersten studies:
• There is little significant improvement following root surface instrumentation of shallow pockets.
• Shallow pockets lose some clinical attachment after instrumentation.
• Pockets of 4-6mm show average probing depth reductions of about 1mm and 0.5mm gain of attachment after treatment.
• Deep pockets show average probing depth reductions of about 2mm and 1mm gain of attachment after treatment.

Summary

This chapter has reviewed the aims of non-surgical treatment as well as the clinical outcomes that have been documented in longitudinal clinical trials. These outcomes should be regarded as the likely consequences of non-surgical treatment. It is essential, however, that the clinician appreciates that there are additional confounding factors that will have a significant effect on the outcome of treatment. These factors must be assessed on an individual patient basis, including:
• patient motivation
• patient compliance
• medical risk factors
• local risk factors

Table 1-2 **Principal conclusions and clinical outcomes following non-surgical treatment of incisors, canines and premolars in patients with moderate and advanced chronic periodontitis.**

Moderately advanced periodontitis (average probing depths 4-7mm)	Advanced chronic periodontitis (probing depths up to 12mm)
• Plaque scores were reduced from 70% to less than 12% within 1 month.	• Significant reductions in plaque scores resulted in 0.5mm reduction in probing depths.
• Bleeding scores were reduced from 90% to 15% over a period of 5 months, but only after the instrumentation phase of treatment had been completed.	• Instrumentation resulted in a further 1.2mm reduction in probing depths.
• Bleeding on probing was encountered more often in deeper residual pockets than in shallow pockets.	• Periodontal status improved during a period of 6-9 months following treatment.
• Probing depths were reduced by approximately 0.5mm after the hygiene phase. The total mean reduction of probing depths after instrumentation was approximately 1.5mm.	• Deep residual pockets were more likely to bleed than shallow pockets.
• More pocket depth reduction and gain of attachment was seen in the initial pockets of >6mm than in those of 4.0–5.5mm.	• Sites with deep probing depths showed more gain of attachment, gingival recession and ultimately, deeper residual probing depths than sites with shallow probing depths.
• Mean gingival recession was 1.5mm one year after the commencement of treatment was started although most of this recession occurred during the first 2-3 months.	
• Most of the clinical improvement occurred within 5 months of treatment.	
• Ultrasonic instrumentation was much quicker than hand instrumentation. There were no differences in clinical efficacy between the two methods.	

(After Badersten, et al. 1981; 1984)

- genetic predisposition to periodontal disease
- the nature of the bacterial challenge.

It is widely recognised that smoking is one of the most prevalent risk factors for periodontal diseases. The magnitude of the clinical change following periodontal treatment in smokers is inferior to the clinical outcome in ex-smokers and those who have never smoked. None of the studies that have been reported in this chapter recognised the potential influence of smoking on chronic periodontitis and its treatment.

Conclusions of Clinical Importance

- The aim of root surface instrumentation is to remove endotoxins and the biofilm from root surfaces.
- As much subgingival calculus as possible should be removed from root surfaces, but some small residual deposits may be compatible with healing.
- Full-mouth disinfection can be used to provide intensive treatment over two visits within 24–48 hours.
- Pockets heal by resolution of inflammation and the formation of a long junctional epithelium.
- Deep pockets show greater reduction of probing depths following treatment than shallow pockets.

Further Reading

Badersten A, Nilveus R, Egelberg J. Effect of nonsurgical periodontal therapy. I. Moderately advanced periodontitis. J Clin Periodontol 1981;8:57-72.

Badersten A, Nilveus R, Egelberg J. Effect of nonsurgical periodontal therapy. II. Severely advanced periodontitis. J Clin Periodontol 1984;11:63-76.

Cercek JF, Kiger RD, Garrett S, Egelberg J. Relative effects of plaque control and instrumentation on the clinical parameters of human periodontal disease. J Clin Periodontol 1983;10:46-56.

Hung H-C, Douglass C-W. Meta-analysis of the effect of scaling and root planing, surgical treatment and antibiotic therapies on periodontal probing depth and attachment loss. J Clin Periodontol 2002;29:975-986.

Jenkins WMM, Said SH, Radvar M, Kinane DF. Effect of subgingival scaling during supportive therapy. J Clin Periodontol 2000;27:590-596.

Chapter 2

Hygiene Phase Therapy

Aims

To provide a comprehensive overview of the methods that are available for the mechanical and chemical control of dental plaque.

Outcome

After reading this chapter the practitioner should:
- be aware of the range of toothbrush designs and interdental cleaning aids that are available
- understand the indications for using chemical plaque control
- have knowledge of the range of generic mouth rinses that are available for chemical plaque control.

Plaque Control Programmes

Homecare, plaque control programmes and hygiene phase therapy are crucial components of non-surgical periodontal therapy. Programmes should be based on individual patient needs in order to achieve a level of plaque control that is compatible with a stable periodontium. It is, however, unrealistic to expect patients to achieve a plaque-free dentition. Indeed, many clinical studies have confirmed that most patients, even with intensive hygiene phase therapy and regular re-enforcement of plaque control measures, will still have about 10-15% of tooth surfaces with residual plaque deposits. For the vast majority of patients with chronic periodontitis, this standard of tooth cleaning may be found to be acceptable.

Clinical trials in the 1980s confirmed that plaque control may be taught effectively in two 15 minute appointments (Table 2-1). It is important that sufficient time is dedicated specifically to the hygiene phase of therapy so that patients appreciate fully that they have the key role to play in the management of their periodontal disease. This role often necessitates significant behavioural and attitude changes with respect to oral healthcare practices. In order to achieve this, patients must be made aware that they are different from the general population with respect to their susceptibility to periodontitis and, con-

Table 2-1 **Typical, two-visit plaque control programme as a component of hygiene phase therapy.**

First visit (15 minutes)	Second visit (15 minutes)
Provide dental health information including, for smokers, the effects of nicotine on oral health	Ask smokers if they are ready to quit and where appropriate provide smoking cessation advice
Disclose and score plaque	Disclose and score plaque and compare to previous score
Advice on the selection of a toothbrush and give instructions in toothbrushing	Identify any problems with tooth brushing and the use of interdental aids. If necessary, reinforce or change advice
Instructions on interdental cleaning	Professional prophylaxis to remove residual stained plaque
Professional prophylaxis to remove residual stained plaque	Always be positive and praise the patient's efforts

sequently, they must achieve exceptionally high standards of homecare if treatment is to succeed.

Mechanical plaque control

Plaque control refers to the removal of plaque from tooth surfaces and gingival tissues, and prevention of new microbial growth. Effective plaque control results in resolution of gingival inflammation and is fundamentally important in all periodontal therapy. Periodontal treatment performed in the absence of plaque control is certain to fail, resulting in disease progression or recurrence. Mechanical plaque control is performed using toothbrushes, toothpaste and other cleaning aids. Plaque control programmes should be tailored to the requirements of individual patients, addressing their local risk factors at the whole mouth, tooth and site levels (see book 1 in this series, *Understanding Periodontal Diseases: Assessment and Diagnostic Procedure in Practice*).

Manual Toothbrushes

Conventional, manual toothbrushes vary in design and size, and the type of brush used is a matter of personal preference (Fig 2-1). Bristles are generally

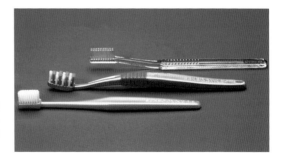

Fig 2-1 A small number of the wide range of manual toothbrushes that are available on the market.

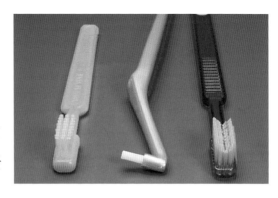

Fig 2-2 Specialist toothbrushes: (left to right) a child's toothbrush, a single tufted toothbrush and an orthodontic toothbrush used to clean around the components of fixed orthodontic appliances.

made of nylon, which is relatively flexible, resistant to fracture and does not become saturated with water. Bristles are arranged in tufts, and round-ended bristles cause fewer scratches on the gingiva than flat-ended bristles do. Softer bristles have greater flexibility, and have been shown to reach further interproximally and subgingivally. Hard bristles are more likely to result in gingival trauma. However, the technique and the force applied when brushing are more important determinants of plaque removal capability and gingival trauma than the hardness of the bristles themselves. With use, toothbrushes show signs of wear and flattening of bristles, and should be replaced approximately every three months. A typical, conventional, manual toothbrush is likely to conform to the following standards:
• brush head dimensions – 1.5-2.5cm long and 0.15-0.75cm wide
• four rows of "bristles" of medium texture and made from nylon polymer filaments of 10-12mm length.

Specialist toothbrushes are available for certain patients and specific clinical indications (Fig 2-2):

- *children's toothbrushes* - which have a reduced head size and a more bulky, easier-to-grip handle
- *single tufted toothbrushes (interspace brushes)* - which can be used in areas that are inaccessible to a conventional brush, e.g. sites of gingival recession, furcations and large interdental spaces
- *orthodontic toothbrushes* - which have a V-shaped indentation along the head of bristles to accommodate the components of fixed orthodontic appliances
- *denture brushes* – which may be used with partial or complete dentures. They usually have a dual-purpose head with tapered bristles that are much firmer than those of a conventional toothbrush.

Powered Toothbrushes

The brush heads of powered toothbrushes (Fig 2-3) tend to be more compact than those of their manual counterparts - a feature that facilitates interproximal brushing and cleaning of, in particular, posterior teeth. Bundles of bristles are arranged in rows in a rectangular head or in a circular pattern

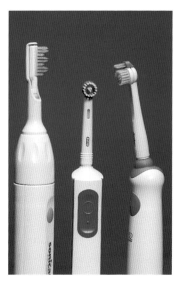

Fig 2-3 Three powered toothbrushes with different handle and brush head designs. The brushes with circular arrangements of bristles operate with an oscillating motion whereas the traditional design of brush head operates with a side-to-side or back and forth motion.

mounted in a round head. Some brushes have single, compact tufts, which are specifically designed for interproximal cleaning. The traditional design of brush head operates with a side-to-side or back and forth motion. Circular heads have an oscillating motion.

Powered brushes have previously been considered particularly beneficial for special needs patients, patients with fixed orthodontic appliances, and those who are hospitalised or institutionalised and who may need a third-party/carer to assist with toothbrushing. It is now more generally accepted that powered brushes may be advantageous for a much wider group of patients who might otherwise be unable to achieve an "acceptable" standard of plaque control. Numerous studies have confirmed that, for most patients, powered brushes are more effective than manual toothbrushes. This may be

Fig 2-4a The Bass method of toothbrushing (for explanation of technique see text); **b** The Charters' method of toothbrushing. This technique involves placement of the bristles at a 45° angle to the long axis of the tooth but, unlike the Bass technique, the bristles are pointed towards the occlusal surface of

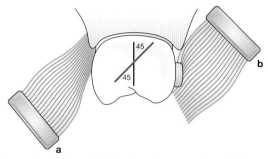

the tooth. This technique may be particularly useful for cleaning around orthodontic brackets in patients undergoing fixed appliance therapy.

because of better mechanical cleaning, although the novelty of using a powered toothbrush may also improve compliance, especially in children.

Contemporary designs of powered toothbrushes have a number of special features that enhance their use:
• timing mechanisms
• easy start features which increase the brushing force over the first few occasions of use
• dual-speed options
• programmable pacers that provide feedback to signal the amount of time that has been spent in one part (quadrant) of the mouth.

Toothpastes

Toothpastes are used as aids for cleaning tooth surfaces and contain abrasives (e.g. silica), water, preservatives, flavouring, colouring, detergents and therapeutic agents (e.g. fluoride). Abrasives (approximately 20-40% of the content) enhance plaque removal, but may result in damage to the tooth surface if there is overzealous brushing. Smokers' toothpastes and tooth powders contain significantly higher proportions of abrasives and their use is not recommended. Chemotherapeutic agents (e.g. chlorhexidine) may be added to toothpastes. These agents are discussed in more detail later in this section.

Toothbrushing techniques

The majority of patients use a "horizontal scrub" technique, which does not clean effectively around gingival margins and can lead to tooth wear. When brushing, a systematic approach is essential, and all accessible surfaces of all teeth should be cleaned thoroughly. The Bass technique is useful for the majority of patients with or without periodontal disease (Fig 2-4). The Charters' method is useful for gentle gingival cleaning, particularly during healing immediately after periodontal surgery and for patients with necrotising gingivitis in whom the painful symptoms have resolved.

Bass Technique
- The toothbrush is placed at the gingival margin, with bristles orientated at 45° to the long axis of the tooth, pointing in an apical direction.
- Short vibratory strokes with light pressure are applied to the brush so that the bristles are not dislodged (the bristles reach interproximally and approximately 1mm subgingivally, resulting in gingival blanching).
- After about 20 strokes, the brush is repositioned to clean the next group of teeth.

The Charters' Method
- Toothbrush is placed on the tooth with the bristles orientated at 45° to the long axis of the tooth, pointing in a coronal direction, such that the sides of the bristles are against the gingival tissues.
- A short back and forth vibratory motion is applied so that the sides of the bristles flex against the gingival margin.

Interproximal Cleaning Aids

Interproximal areas are particularly susceptible to plaque accumulation and subsequent attachment loss because toothbrushing does not always remove plaque from these surfaces. Additional cleaning aids are, therefore, required.

Dental Floss and Tape
Floss is usually made from nylon, and is available as a twisted or untwisted multifilament, with or without a coating of wax (wax facilitates passage beyond the contact point), as a thread or in tape form. Floss made from expanded polytetrafluoroethylene (Teflon) materials that do not fray is also available. The plaque removal capabilities of different types of floss do not vary significantly from each other. About 45cm of dental floss should be wrapped around the middle fingers of each hand, leaving about 3-4cm stretched tightly between the thumbs, or thumb and first finger of each hand so that it can be eased carefully past the proximal contact point. The floss should be moved carefully up and down the proximal surface of each tooth, from just below the contact area to just below the gingival margin. Floss

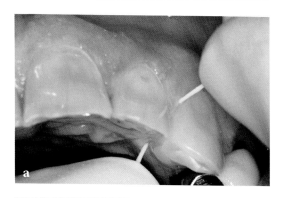

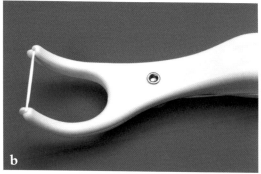

Fig 2-5a Correct application of dental floss to clean interproximally beneath contact areas; **b** Some patients may find this technique to be particularly difficult to master and may benefit from the use of a floss holder; **c** Superfloss is particularly useful for cleaning between natural teeth and the components of a bridge, particularly beneath pontics.

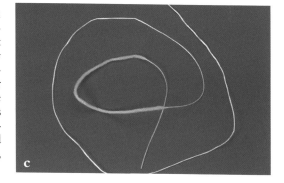

holders, which stretch the floss between two plastic supports, may be useful for patients with limited manual dexterity (Fig 2-5).

Dental tape is essentially a thicker, flatter form of floss that comprises a single

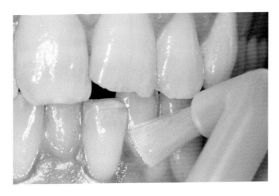

Fig 2-6 An interspace brush is useful for cleaning inaccessible areas including root surfaces affected by gingival recession and the interproximal surfaces of teeth when adjacent teeth are absent.

fibre that reduces the likelihood of fraying or shredding. Tape, like floss may be impregnated with active ingredients such as chlorhexidine and fluoride.

Superfloss
Superfloss is specifically designed to clean beneath bridge pontics and comprises three parts (Fig 2-5c):
- one end is coated with wax to facilitate threading beneath the components of the bridge
- a spongy central section for cleaning beneath pontics
- a "tail" of conventional floss for use interdentally between retainers and natural teeth.

Interspace Brushes (Fig 2-6)
Interspace or single-tufted brushes have just one tuft of bristles. These are especially useful for cleaning:
- proximal surfaces of teeth when adjacent teeth are absent
- distal surfaces of the most posterior remaining tooth
- the lingual surfaces of mandibular teeth
- around orthodontic appliances
- areas of gingival recession
- areas of crowding with instanding teeth that are missed by a regular toothbrush
- tooth/root concavities and incipient (class I) furcation lesions
- exposed portions of implants.

Interdental Brushes (Fig 2-7)
Interdental brushes are conical or tube-like brushes ("bottle brushes") made

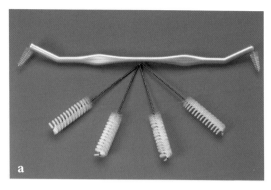

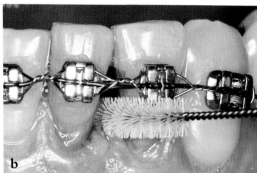

Fig 2-7a A range of interdental brushes that are available; **b** An interdental brush being used to clean interproximally between mandibular incisors in a patient undergoing fixed appliance orthodontic therapy.

of bristles mounted on a twisted metal wire handle. They are available in many different designs and sizes, and may be used to clean:

- interproximally, particularly in locations where there is loss of the interdental papilla and there is sufficient room for the brush
- subgingivally
- in class II and class III furcations
- around implant restorations (the wire handle being plastic-coated to prevent scratching of the implant surface).

Woodsticks (Fig 2-8)
Woodsticks are triangular in cross-section, made of soft birch wood, and are used to dislodge plaque and debris from accessible interdental sites in anterior teeth. There is a risk that the wood may splinter and there is a tendency for self-inflicted trauma unless patients have been instructed very carefully in their use. They are not suitable for use in young children.

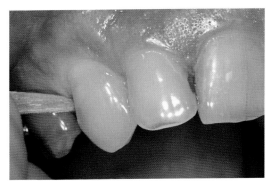

Fig 2-8 Correct use of a wood stick to dislodge plaque and debris from an interdental site between anterior teeth. Note that wood sticks have to be used with extreme care and patients must be reminded that the flat base of the stick must always be adjacent to the gingival tissues.

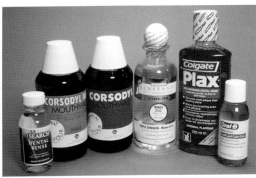

Fig 2-9 A small number of the vast range of commercially available mouth rinses that may be used for chemical plaque control. Many patients, however, use these products simply as a means of "freshening their breath".

Chemical Plaque Control (Fig 2-9)

Chemical agents have been incorporated into mouth rinses and toothpastes with the objective of inhibiting the formation of plaque and calculus (Table 2-2). Antiplaque agents may, therefore, have a significant clinical effect of resolving an established gingivitis.

Cationic agents
Chlorhexidine digluconate
Chlorhexidine is frequently used as a mouth rinse (0.2% or 0.12% w/v). The compound can also be applied as a gel (Fig 1-5), and has been incorporated into:
- chewing gum
- floss
- sprays
- slow-release devices for controlled release of chlorhexidine directly into pockets

Table 2-2 **Examples of commercially available mouth rinses that are designed for chemical plaque control.**

Mouthrinse	Main active agent	Manufacturer
Sensitive™	cetylpyridinium chloride	Boots
Complete Care™	cetylpyridinium chloride	Macleans
Oracle™	cetylpyridinium chloride	Safeway
Sensodyne™ Gentle	cetylpyridinium chloride	GlaxoSmithKline
Dentimint Total Care™	cetylpyridinium chloride	McBride
Aquafresh™	cetylpyridinium chloride	GlaxoSmithKline
Antiplaque™	cetylpyridinium chloride	Oral B
Coolmint/Freshmint	cetylpyridinium chloride	Tesco
Dentyl pH™	cetylpyridinium chloride, triclosan	Fresh Breath Ltd.
Corsodyl™	chlorhexidine 0.2%	GlaxoSmithKline
Chlorohex™	chlorhexidine 0.12%	Colgate
Listerine™	thymol, zinc chloride	Pfizer
Plax™	triclosan, sodium lauryl sulphate, PVA/MA co-polymer	Colgate

- periodontal packs.

At low concentrations, chlorhexidine is bacteriostatic, but at high concentrations, it is bactericidal. The mode of action of chlorhexidine in killing bacteria is dependent upon the agent having access to cell walls. Electrostatic forces facilitate this, since chlorhexidine is positively charged, whilst the phosphate and carboxyl groups of bacterial cell walls carry negative charges. Binding causes disruption of the osmotic barrier and interference with membrane transport.

Rinsing with chlorhexidine reduces the number of bacteria in saliva by between 50% and 90%. A maximum reduction of 95% occurs around five days, after which the numbers increase gradually to maintain an overall reduction of 70-80% at 40 days.

An important property of chlorhexidine is its *substantivity*, that is, the retention in the mouth and subsequent release from oral structures. After a one-minute oral rinse of 10ml of chlorhexidine 0.2%, approximately 30% of the drug is retained, and within 15 seconds of rinsing, half will have bonded to receptor molecules.

Chlorhexidine mouth rinses and gels should be used in the short-term until toothbrushing and use of interdental aids are able to remove plaque effectively. For example:
• after periodontal surgery in the reduction of postoperative infection, pain and inflammation
• in the management of periodontal problems as part of a palliative care programme
• to help prevent drug-induced gingival overgrowth
• to help prevent secondary infection in the management of necrotising ulcerative gingivitis and periodontitis
• for patients provided with fixed orthodontic appliances or intermaxillary fixation devices
• to help reduce superinfection of gingival ulcerative conditions, e.g. viral infections and erosive lichen planus (desquamative gingivitis).

The main unwanted effects of chlorhexidine are:
• staining of the teeth, calculus, restorations and the tongue (Fig 2-10)
• taste disturbances.

Chlorhexidine should, therefore, only used for short periods (two to three weeks). Toothpaste components called anionic surfactants interact with chlorhexidine activity and lower its effective delivery to the tooth surface. It is therefore, not recommended that chlorhexidine be used before or imme-

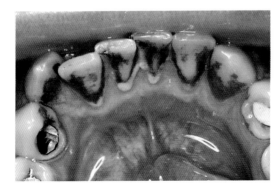

Fig 2-10 Characteristic chlorhexidine staining of anterior teeth and calculus.

diately following toothbrushing. If toothpaste has been used before rinsing, paste should be rinsed away before using the chlorhexidine mouth rinse.

Quaternary ammonium compounds (QACs)
Examples are cetylpyridinium chloride (CPC) (often combined with domiphen bromide), benzalconium chloride and benzethonium chloride. These substances have a net positive charge, which reacts with the negatively charged phosphate groups on bacterial cell walls. The walls are disrupted, resulting in increased permeability and loss of cell contents.

Studies suggest that CPC 0.05% (with or without domiphen bromide) and benzethonium chloride causes a reduction in plaque of between 25% and 35%, but with less obvious effects on gingival inflammation. CPC (0.1%) is also marketed as a pre-brushing rinse.

Phenols
Phenols exert a non-specific antibacterial action, which is dependent upon the ability of the drug, in the non-ionized form, to penetrate the lipid components of bacterial cell walls. Phenolic compounds may also exhibit anti-inflammatory properties, which may result from their ability to inhibit neutrophil chemotaxis, the neutralisation of neutrophil-derived superoxide anions and the production of prostaglandin synthetase.

Listerine™
Listerine™ is an over-the-counter antiplaque agent that contains thymol (0.06%), eucalyptol (0.09%), methyl salicylate (0.06%) and methanol (0.04%) in 16.9% alcohol. Twice daily rinsing with 20ml of Listerine™ as a supplement to normal oral hygiene produces a 35% reduction in plaque and gingivitis scores.

Triclosan™
Triclosan™ is a bisphenol, non-ionic germicide with a broad spectrum of activity against gram-positive and gram-negative bacteria and fungi. The compound adsorbs on to the lipid portion of the bacterial cell membrane and blocks lipid synthesis. At low concentrations, Triclosan interferes with vital transport mechanisms in bacteria. A concentration of between 0.1% and 0.2% is suitably efficacious with minimal side effects. Activity is enhanced when the compound is combined with zinc citrate or incorporated into a copolymer of methoxyethylene and maleic acid. The copolymer increases the substantivity of Triclosan™ and acts as a reservoir.

Plax™

Plax™ rinse is a combination of anionic and ionic surfactants including sodium lauryl sulphate and polysorbate 20. Triclosan 0.3% and a methoxyethylene and maleic acid copolymer have been added to the rinse that is now marketed as an anti-plaque product.

Sanguinarine

Sanguinarine is a benzophenathridine alkaloid structure obtained by alcoholic extraction from the bloodroot plant Sanguinaria candensis. Antibacterial properties of sanguinarine are thought to be due to its ability to suppress the activity of intracellular bacterial enzymes, possibly through oxidation of thiol groups. The extract has been incorporated into a mouth rinse and toothpaste, and 0.03% is the most frequently evaluated concentration. The anti-plaque efficacy is low when compared to that of chlorhexidine. The main advantage of sanguinarine over chlorhexidine is the relative absence of unwanted effects. A mild to moderate burning sensation in the mouth and mild sloughing of the oral mucosa have been reported.

Heavy metal salts

Salts of zinc, tin and copper are reported to inhibit the growth of dental plaque and impede calculus formation.

Zinc salts

Zinc salts possess antiplaque activity although generally it is lower than that of chlorhexidine. Zinc citrate and chloride are frequently incorporated into toothpaste. Zinc salts exhibit good substantivity, with 30% of zinc retained in the mouth after toothbrushing with a 0.5% zinc citrate toothpaste. The activity of both zinc citrate and Triclosan™ is enhanced when the products are used in combination.

Tin salts

The suggested antibacterial mechanisms of tin ions are thought to be mediated through their ability to bind to lipotechoic acid present on the surfaces of gram-positive bacteria. The net surface charge of the organism is therefore reversed and the adsorption of the bacteria on tooth surfaces is reduced. The accumulation of tin in bacteria may alter their metabolism and other physicochemical characteristics. Stannous salts cause staining of the teeth and the tongue, although the stain is easily removed using prophylaxis paste.

Enzymes

Research into the use of enzymes as antiplaque agents has been largely discontinued. One enzyme system that is currently available is the lactoperoxidase-hypothiocyanite system.

Lactoperoxidase-hypothiocyanite
Certain oral bacteria are known to produce hydrogen peroxide (H_2O_2) by the oxidation of the glycolytic enzyme $NADH_2$ by $NADH_2$ oxidase. This H_2O_2 either oxidizes another $NADH_2$ molecule or is inactivated by the enzyme catalase. When the level of H_2O_2 in saliva is increased, it assists lactoperoxidase in the oxidation of thiocyanate (SCN^-) to produce the hypothiocyanite ion ($OSCN^-$). The latter interferes with the redox mechanisms of cells by upsetting the $NADH_2$- $NADPH_2$ balance. The production is achieved by introducing a further enzyme system involving amyloglucosidase and glucose oxidase. This system is the basis for the production of the commercially available toothpaste Zendium^{TM} (Oral B, UK). In addition to amyloglycosidase (1.2% w/w) and glucose oxidase (1.0% w/w), Zendium contains potassium thiocyanite (0.2% w/w) and sodium fluoride (0.26%).

Key Points of Clinical Importance

- Complete removal of plaque is an unrealistic aim and plaque control programmes should be tailored to the individual needs of patients.
- For any individual, the level of plaque control achieved should be consistent with oral health. That is, the threshold level required to resolve inflammation varies from patient to patient.
- The hygiene phase of non-surgical treatment involves instruction in the use of toothbrushes, a toothbrushing technique and the use of interdental cleaning aids.
- Studies have shown that powered toothbrushes may be marginally more efficient than conventional toothbrushes but this may, in part, be a result of the novelty effect of using a new product.
- There is a wide range of interdental aids available on the market and these should also be carefully tailored to the individual needs of patients.
- There is a wide range of mouth rinses available for chemical control of plaque. Such products should, whenever possible, be for short-term use until a patient is able to reintroduce or master adequate mechanical plaque control.
- There are few reasons to recommend mouth rinses for patients who perform adequate plaque control.
- Research suggests that chlorhexidine is the most effective agent for chemical plaque control, but it should not be used within an hour of toothbrushing.

Further Reading

Chapple ILC, Gilbert AD. Understanding Periodontal Diseases: Assessment and Diagnostic Procedures in Practice. London: Quintessence, 2002.

Heasman PA, McCracken GI. Clinical evidence for the safety and efficacy of powered toothbrushes. Adv Dent Res 2002;16:1-7.

Heasman PA, McCracken GI. Powered toothbrushes: A review of clinical trials. J Clin Periodontol 1999;26:407-420.

Heasman PA, Seymour RA. Pharmacological control of periodontal disease. I. Anti plaque agents. J Dent 1994;22:323-335.

Chapter 3
Instruments and Instrumentation

Aim

The aim of this chapter is to describe a range of instruments used for the non-surgical management of periodontal disease.

Outcome

After reading this chapter the reader should be able to identify the various types of instruments and have an understanding of the purpose of each periodontal instrument, and its advantages and disadvantages in different situations.

Introduction

The instruments used for periodontal non-surgical management can be divided into of two main categories:
- hand instruments
- powered instruments (sonic scalers, ultrasonic scalers and air-abrasive devices).

Hand Instruments

There are many groups of instruments that are used for scaling procedures. Each instrument is designed for use in a specific area of the mouth. An instrument can be categorised by:
- whether it is to be used for supragingival or subgingival instrumentation
- whether it is a universal or area/tooth specific instrument.

Scaling instruments fall into the general categories of:
- chisels
- trihedral scalers
- hoes
- files
- curettes.

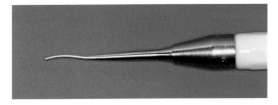

Fig 3-1 The chisel scaler is a straight instrument that curves slightly as the blade extends from the shank.

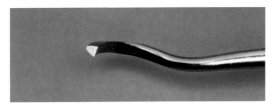

Fig 3-2 The working end of trihedral scaler is triangular in cross section.

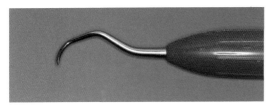

Fig 3-3 For lower anterior teeth a mini-sickle scaler has a tighter curve at the instruments working end.

Chisel Scaler or Push Scaler (Guy's G1 or G2, Cushings or Watch-Spring)
The chisel scaler is a straight instrument that curves slightly as the blade extends from the shank (Fig 3-1). The end of the blade is flat, with a straight cutting edge that is bevelled at 45°. It is available in different widths and is used with a controlled push stroke from the labial aspect of the lower anterior teeth to remove interproximal and lingual supragingival calculus. It should only be used where there is sufficient embrasure space or gingival trauma will result. It may be used subgingivally where the interdental papillae have lost attachment. A mouth mirror should always be used to protect the tongue and the floor of the mouth.

Trihedral Scalers (H6, H7, G3, G4, J1 and H5)
The working end of trihedral scalers is triangular in cross-section (Fig 3-2). It is designed so that its lower border does not damage gingival tissue. There are two blades, one either side of the superior surface, which end in a point. The blades curve in a lateral plane allowing them to engage the tooth surface. The shank may be straight or contra-angled. There are two main types of trihedral scalers: sickle scalers and jacquette scalers (G3, G4, J1 and H5).

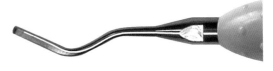

Fig 3-4 Periodontal hoe used for root surface instrumentation

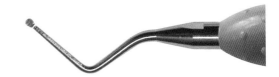

point 1

point 2

Fig 3-5 When using a periodontal hoe a two-point contact must be maintained.

Fig 3-6 A periodontal file has multiple straight cutting edges.

Sickle scalers (H6 and H7) are principally used for the removal of supragingival calculus or for subgingival calculus that is located just below the gingival margin. For lower anterior teeth a minisickle scaler has a tighter curve at the instrument's working end that contours more efficiently (Fig 3-3).

Periodontal Hoes
Periodontal hoes (Fig 3-4) have variously angled shanks with a functional "lip" at the end. The single blade is bevelled. Hoes can be used on all tooth surfaces and are primarily used for subgingival scaling and root surface instrumentation. Periodontal hoes are used with a "pull action" parallel to the long axis of the tooth. It is important that a two-point contact is maintained (Fig 3-5) throughout the instrument stroke. Care must be taken to avoid gouging of the cementum with the corners of the blade. These instruments are difficult to sharpen, although tungsten carbide hoes are durable and require less frequent sharpening. There are four instruments, which are designed to enable the mesial, distal, buccal and lingual surfaces to be instrumented (TC 210, 211, 212, and 213). Table 3-1 shows the advantages and disadvantages of periodontal hoes.

Table 3-1 **Advantages and disadvantages of periodontal hoes.**

Advantages	Disadvantages
Only four types, so instrument selection is easy	Only one-point root surface contact (poor efficiency)
Rigid shanks result in easier removal of tenacious calculus	Too wide for narrow pockets
Good for wide pockets	Do not contour root surface
	Increased risk of hard and soft tissue trauma due to sharp corners
	Tungsten carbide tips require special sharpening kits
	Blade at 90° to shank (not ideal)
	Not designed for ease of access to posterior teeth
	Finger rest difficult to obtain local to point of action

Periodontal Files (Hirschfeld 3/7, 5/11 and 9/10)
A periodontal file (Fig 3-6) is an instrument that has multiple, straight cutting edges at the working end of the instrument. There are two main indications for using the periodontal file to facilitate calculus removal. The first is for the removal of burnished calculus deposits that have previously been "over instrumented" and have become smooth. Burnished calculus commonly results from sonic/ultrasonic instrumentation and is difficult to remove because the cutting edge of the instrument tends to slide over the smooth surface. A file is used to roughen the surface of the burnished deposit so that it can then be removed by another instrument. The second indication is for "crushing" calculus making it easier to remove with a curette. Each file is designed for use on a single tooth surface: mesial, distal, lingual and palatal. Diamond tipped files make furcation instrumentation much easier.

Curettes
There are two main categories of curette:
• universal
• area-specific.

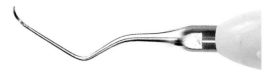

Fig 3-7 A universal curette is used for subgingival instrumentation.

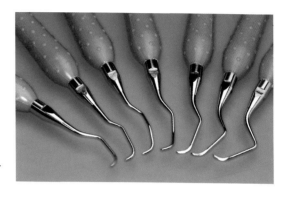

Fig 3-8 Gracey curettes, area-specific instruments.

Universal Curettes (Columbia 2R/2L; Columbia 13/14; Langers 1/2; Langers 5/6, and Langers)

A universal curette (Fig 3-7) is an instrument with a rounded back and rounded toe. Universal curettes have two parallel cutting edges at the working end. Usually curettes are paired as a double-ended instrument and can be applied to all tooth surfaces in both the anterior and posterior parts of the mouth. There are numerous designs of universal curette. In selecting a universal curette for a particular task, the operator should consider the design characteristics of the working end and functional shank. The universal curette is used throughout the entire mouth for the removal of both supragingival and subgingival calculus. Although the cutting edges are several millimetres long, adaptation of the universal curette to the tooth surface is achieved by placing the distal 2 to 3mm of the blade in the appropriate working relationship next to the tooth surface.

Area-specific curettes/site specific curettes

Area- or site-specific curettes are designed for use in particular anatomical areas of the mouth. The most commonly used specific curettes are Gracey curettes (Fig 3-8) that were designed by Dr Clayton Gracey in the 1930s. The name "area-specific" signifies that each curette can be applied only to

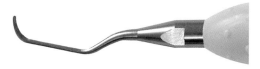

Fig 3-9 Gracey curettes have an angled working end.

certain surfaces, and for this reason, a complete set of curettes is needed to instrument the entire dentition. Area-specific curettes were intended to provide access for scaling and root surface instrumentation on root surfaces with deep pockets (>5mm, hence the term "Gracey after-five" curettes is used) and attachment loss without causing trauma to the pocket epithelium. Gracey curettes are characterised by their unique blade features and long flexible shanks. Some instruments are designed with complex bends that dramatically improve operator access to complex root morphology (Fig 3-9).

The original Gracey Series contains fourteen curettes although rarely are all fourteen curettes used in practice. The curettes are available as single-ended or double-ended versions, the double-ended instruments having "mirror image" blades. A standard set that may be used to access all tooth surfaces (Fig 3-8) would include:
- Gracey 1-2 – for all surfaces of anterior teeth
- Gracey 7-8 – for facial and lingual surfaces of molars and premolars
- Gracey 13-14 – for distal surfaces of molars and premolars
- Gracey 15-16 – for mesial surfaces of molars and premolars (or 11-12)
- Gracey 17-18 – for distal surfaces of molar teeth of difficult access.

The working end of the Gracey curette is designed differently from that of the universal curette or sickle scalers. The face of the blade is machined onto the Gracey instrument at a 70° angle to the lower or terminal shank. The opposite cutting edge is machined off in the manufacturing process leaving one cutting edge on each end of the instrument to avoid soft tissue trauma during use. Viewed in cross section, the cutting blade is the lower edge of the instrument.

The cutting edge can be readily identified by visually comparing the angle of the face of the blade to the lower shank and therefore selecting the correct "lower cutting edge". Furthermore, if the face of the blade is examined to compare the curvature of the two sides of the working end, then the "longer" or "convex" curved blade is selected. The application of the prin-

Table 3-2 **Universal versus Gracey curettes.**

Universal	Gracey
One design for all areas and surfaces	Designed for specific teeth and surfaces
Face of blade at 90° to shank	Face of blade at 70° to shank
Two cutting edges	One cutting edge only
Curved in one direction only	Curved in two planes; up and to the side
Shorter shanks	Long curved shanks
Shanks are flexible but less so than the Gracey curettes	Flexible shanks reduce finger strain and root surface damage

ciples of blade design allows the identification of the cutting edge of any of the Gracey Series curettes. A set of Gracey curettes called "mini five" curettes has been designed to enable access to narrow pockets; their numbering is the same as for the "after five" series. Table 3-2 demonstrates the differences between Universal and Gracey curettes.

Recommended Protocol for Root Surface Instrumentation (RSI)

- Re-check probing depths/bleeding/deposits.
- Apply local anaesthesia.
- Chlorhexidine rinse (0.2%) will reduce microbial contamination in aerosol by 90%.
- Explore root surface thoroughly with World Health Organization (WHO) probe or similar (e.g. "Old Dominican University" (ODU) explorer - see below).
- Use ultrasonic scaler (see protocol below).
- Re-explore with WHO/ODU explorer.
- Use hand instruments for fine tactile work (e.g. Gracey curettes).
- Re-check with explorer and repeat as necessary.
- Finish with ultrasonic instrument to irrigate the pockets.

Mechanised Instruments

Mechanised scalers are power-driven units that convert electrical energy to mechanical energy to remove supragingival and subgingival calculus deposits

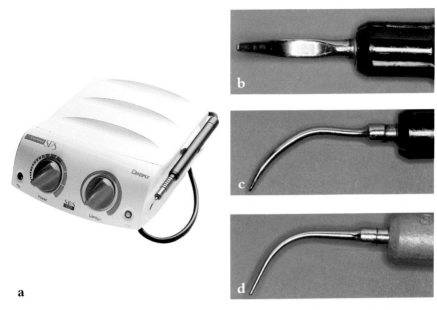

Fig 3-10 a Magnetostrictive (Cavitron) scaler manufactured by Dentsply; **b** beavertail tip used for removal of heavy calculus deposits; **c** universal tip used for moderate supra- and subgingival calculus deposits; **d** precision(slimline) tip used to provide best access to deep pockets and furcation areas.

from the teeth and bacterial plaque from periodontal pockets. Ultrasonic instruments were introduced for scaling in 1955 and are now commonly used for periodontal treatment. The two categories of mechanised instruments are ultrasonic units and sonic handpieces; both vibrate at a high frequency using a water-cooled system.

Ultrasonic Units

Ultrasonic units comprise an electric generator, a handpiece, and interchangeable instrument tips. These units work by converting electrical current to mechanical energy in the form of high-frequency vibrations of the instrument tip. Ultrasonic devices operate at frequencies above the audible range; 18,000 to 50,000 cycles per second (18 to 50 kHz) range. There are two types of ultrasonic units:
- magnetostrictive, e.g. Dentsply Cavitron™ (Fig 3-10)
- piezoelectric, e.g. MS Unit (Fig 3-11).

36

Magnetostrictive Units

Magnetostrictive ultrasonic units (Fig 3-10a) are housed in portable units that contain an electric generator and a water control system. The water-cooling system can be connected to the main water supply or a separate portable unit, which can be used to deliver antibacterial medicaments into the periodontal pocket. However, several studies have demonstrated no significant improvement in clinical outcomes, when chlorhexidine is used as an irrigant over water irrigation, because chlorhexidine does not remain within the pocket for long enough to be effective. Most units use removable instrument inserts that fit into the handpiece. The electric generator produces a low-voltage electric current in the handpiece. This current produces a magnetic field in the handpiece that causes the insert to expand and contract along its length and, in turn, causes the insert to vibrate. The pattern of vibration of the tip is elliptical, which means that all sides of the tip are active when adapted to the tooth surface.

Inserts for magnetostrictive units

Modern ultrasonic instrument inserts range in size from large, broad tips to precision thin inserts. Each manufacturing company produces unique instrument inserts for their ultrasonic units. The variety of insert designs varies from company to company, and one manufacturer's tips will not necessarily fit another company's ultrasonic unit. Ultrasonic inserts should be selected in a similar manner to hand instruments. Large, broad working ends (beavertail) are designed to remove heavy supragingival calculus deposits, especially from the lingual aspects of anterior teeth (Fig 3-10b). Medium-sized working ends (universal or sickle: Fig 3-10c) are used to remove moderate supragingival calculus deposits and may be used subgingivally if tissue distension allows for easy insertion of the tip. With this universal application the tips can therefore be used for both anterior and posterior teeth. Precision thin (or slimline) tips (Fig 3-10d) provide the best access to deep pockets and furcation areas and are used to remove subgingival deposits (precision thin ultrasonic tips are similar in diameter to periodontal probes).

Piezoelectric Ultrasonic Units

The piezoelectric ultrasonic (Fig 3-11) device is housed in a portable unit that contains an electric generator and a water control system. The unit may have either a fluid reservoir or tubing used to connect the unit to an external water supply. If a fluid reservoir is available this can be used to irrigate periodontal pockets with an antibacterial medicament. In piezoelectric units the pattern of the vibration of the tip is back and forth, with the two sides of the tip being active.

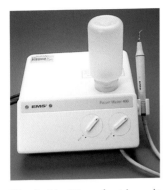

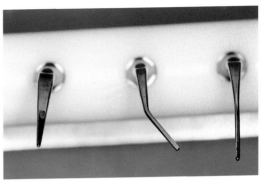

Fig 3-11 Piezoelectric unit manufactured by MS.

Fig 3-12 Piezoelectric tips (from left to right: tip A, tip B, tip P).

Inserts for piezoelectric units

Instrument tips screw directly into the handpiece with the aid of a special tool. The electric generator produces an alternating, high voltage in the handpiece. The voltage produces an electric field in the handpiece that causes the piezo crystals to expand and contract along their diameter, which causes the instrument tip to vibrate. There are a variety of tips available for piezoelectric units (Fig 3-12). Tip A is recommended for supra- and subgingival calculus, tip B is used for deposits on the lingual surface, tip P irrigates subgingival pockets and removes subgingival calculus and tip PS is used for root surface instrumentation.

Sonic Handpieces

Sonic handpieces are mechanised instruments comprising an air-driven handpiece and removable instrument tips. Sonic handpieces (Fig 3-13) use air pressure to create mechanical vibrations that in turn cause the instrument tip to vibrate. The instrument tip of a sonic handpiece vibrates between 3,000 to 8,000 cycles per second (3-8 kHz). Sonic instruments are less efficient in removing calculus deposits than ultrasonic instruments, because the sonic instrument tip vibrates at a slower rate. The slower rate of vibration of the sonic instrument tip results in fewer instrument strokes per second for calculus removal. However, despite this difference, studies have shown that clinical outcomes following sonic and ultrasonic instrumentation for management of chronic periodontitis are equivalent.

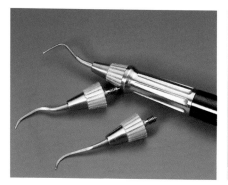 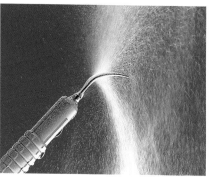

Fig 3-13 Sonic handpiece is an air-driven hand piece.

Fig 3-14 Ultrasonic mist is produced when using the ultrasonic scaler.

Inserts for sonic handpieces
The instrument tips screw directly onto the handpiece with the use of a special tool. Again, the tips are not interchangeable from manufacturer to manufacturer, and most units are limited to standard size instrument tip designs. For this reason, sonic instruments are restricted to the removal of supragingival or subgingival deposits if tissue distension permits easy insertion of the tip. Sonic handpieces cannot be used with antimicrobial solutions as they connect directly to the dental unit and have no ability to accommodate a fluid reservoir.

Air-Abrasive Systems
Air–abrasive systems are relatively new but there is limited research data on the efficacy of these systems. They appear to be more efficient in removal of extrinsic stain, e.g. tea, coffee or tobacco.

Ultrasonic Techniques
- Use a low power setting for most situations. For tenacious calculus, a medium power setting can be used. It is not necessary to use the high power setting; studies have shown that this setting is no more effective than a medium power setting and it may increase the risk of root surface trauma/damage.
- Adjust fluid until a fine mist or a mist with fluid droplets is observed around the instrument tip (Fig 3-14).
- Maintain a light, relaxed grasp.
- Use an intraoral or extraoral finger rest.
- Position the tip with the point directed towards the junctional epithe-

lium and the length of the tip at a 0° to 15° angle to the tooth surface. Apply the point of the instrument tip against the uppermost edge of the deposit.

- A digital action is then used with light pressure; moderate let alone firm pressure decreases the effectiveness of the instrument tip.
- Keep the instrument tip moving at all times, with multiple, light, overlapping strokes to cover the entire tooth surface.

Ultrasonic instrumentation has been shown to be as effective as hand instrumentation and to have several advantages over hand and instrument alternatives (Table 3-3).

Table 3-3 **Hand vs. ultrasonic instrumentation.**

Ultrasonic instrumentation	Hand instrumentation
Several mechanisms of action: cavitation, acoustic turbulence, fluid lavage and mechanical action.	Only one mechanism of action: mechanical action.
Ability to disrupt and destroy bacteria from a distance.	Can remove only what it touches.
Flushing action removes debris and bacteria from pockets.	Some debris remains in pocket to cause irritation to tissue.
Small tip size (0.3-0.6mm).	Large in size (0.76-1.0mm).
Tip has 360° circle of activity and is effective no matter which surface is instrumented.	Only a correctly adapted cutting edge is capable of calculus removal.
Light lateral and relaxed pressure is used for calculus removal.	Moderate to firm lateral pressure is needed for calculus removal.
Relatively little time is needed for calculus removal.	Time needed for calculus removal.
Easily inserted into pockets with minimal distention (stretching) of pocket wall.	Must be positioned apical to deposit resulting in considerable distention of pocket wall.
Limited tissue trauma and faster healing rate.	Tissue trauma and slow healing rate.
Limited cementum removal.	Cementum removal.
No sharpening needed.	Frequent sharpening needed.

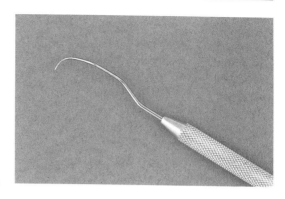

Fig 3-15 The ODU explorer.

Periodontal Explorer

The ODU explorer is available from several manufacturers and is designed with a similar shank pattern to a Gracey 1/2 curette (Fig 3-15). The explorer has a fine tip, which allows easy access to narrow pockets for sensitive root surface exploration (for subgingival deposits, root cracks or grooves).

Repetitive Strain Injury

Clinicians involved in regular use of hand and ultrasonic instrumentation should give careful thought to the use of ergonomically designed instruments to reduce occupational repetitive strain in the hands. This can lead to Carpel Tunnel syndrome (CTS) and other upper body neuropathies, the risk factors for which are discussed in more detail in the second book in this series (*Decision-Making for the Periodontal Team*). Fig 3-16 indicates the areas where pressure points develop. CTS specifically results from inflammation or pressure to the median nerve of the wrist as it passes through the carpel tunnel at the base of the palm of the hand. Symptoms in the hand include:

* tingling
* numbness
* pain.

Metallic hexagonal-shaped instrument handles are thought by some to increase the pressure on important regions within the hand, due to the close "pinch-grip" needed to hold the instruments. The clinical illustrations in Figs 3-17 and 3-18 demonstrate instrumentation that is more ergonomically designed, with thick silicone handles to separate the fingers and facilitate a lighter grip.

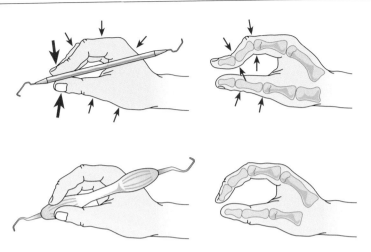

Fig 3-16 Pressure points when undertaking periodontal instrumentation.

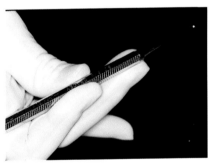

Fig 3-17 Hexagonal-shaped handles should be pinched to ensure a sound grip.

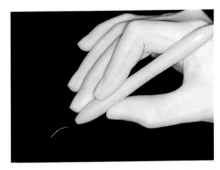

Fig 3-18 An ergonomically designed silicone handle is held lightly.

Conclusions of Clinical Importance

- Recent research has shown that there appears to be no difference in the efficacy of debridement using ultrasonic/sonic and hand instruments.
- With the loss of tactile sense when using an ultrasonic scaler, clinicians may prefer to commence debridement with an ultrasonic scaler and complete the debridement with hand instruments.
- Careful thought should be given to the choice of instruments that will reduce the risk/incidence of repetitive strain injury.

- Antiseptic irrigants have been shown to offer no advantages over water in improving clinical outcomes when powered instruments are used.

Further Reading

Chapple ILC, Walmsley AD, Moscrop H, Saxby MS. Effect of instrument power setting during ultrasonic scaling upon treatment outcome. J Periodontol 1995;66:756-760.

Chapple ILC, Walmsley AD, Moscrop H, Saxby MS. The effect of subgingival irrigation with chlorhexidine during ultrasonic scaling. J Periodontol 1992;63:812-816.

Nield-Gehrig J. Fundamentals of Periodontal Instrumentation, Philadelphia, PA: Lippincott Williams and Watkins, 2000.

Perry D, Beemsterboer P, Carranza F. Techniques and Theory of Periodontal Instrumentation, Philadelphia, PA: WB Saunders Company, 1990.

Trenter SC, Walmsley AD. Ultrasonic dental scaler: associated hazards. J Clin Periodontol 2003;30:95-101.

Tunkel J, Heinecke A, Fleming TF. A systematic review of efficacy of machine-driven and manual subgingival debridment in the treatment of chronic periodontitis. J Clin Periodontol 2002;29:72-81.

Chapter 4
Managing Systemic Risk Factors

Aim

Patients with periodontitis frequently present with one or more systemic conditions that increase their risk of developing periodontitis and which must be considered when planning treatment (Fig 4-1). This chapter aims to provide practical guidance for practitioners in managing the most important and frequently occurring risk factors for periodontitis as part of comprehensive treatment planning.

Outcome

After reading this chapter, the reader should:
- understand the role of risk factor management in periodontal treatment
- be better informed on how to deliver specific risk factor management strategies, in particular, smoking cessation counselling
- understand the importance of close collaboration and team work with other members of the dental team and medical colleagues when treating patients with periodontitis and known risk factors for periodontal disease.

Definitions

The concept of periodontal risk factors, including risk assessment, was described in *Understanding Periodontal Diseases: Assessment and Diagnostic Procedures in Practice*. To recap, a *risk factor* is a factor that increases the probability that a disease may develop in a given individual. Risk factors can be broadly divided into systemic risk factors (subject-based risk factors) or local risk factors (tooth- or site-based risk factors). This chapter will deal specifically with the role of the clinician in managing patients who present with specific systemic risk factors.

Risk Factor Identification

The first step in managing risk factors is to identify precisely which risk factors the patient presents with. This information becomes apparent during history-taking and examination. A full medical history must be recorded,

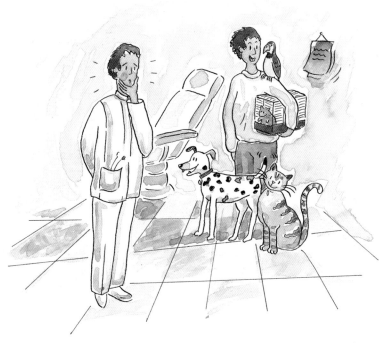

Fig 4-1 "I'm sorry, but genetic testing for gum disease is only done in humans."

including details of ongoing medical treatment, current medications, and whether the patient suffers from any medical condition that might affect the periodontal diagnosis or therapy. History-taking has been covered in detail in *Understanding Periodontal Diseases: Assessment and Diagnostic Procedure in Practice*. From the perspective of risk factor management in periodontics, perhaps the most important considerations are:
- family history
- smoking history
- diabetic status of the patient.

These will be discussed below, together with other systemic risk factors for periodontal disease. Management of risk factors should form an integral part of the treatment of patients with periodontitis as part of a comprehensive therapeutic strategy.

Genetic Risk Factors for Periodontitis

A large body of evidence now supports the theory that genetic factors play an important role in determining susceptibility to periodontitis. We now realise that the host response has a key role in disease pathogenesis and that components of the host response are under genetic control. Both under-activity (hypo-responsiveness) and over-activity (hyper-responsiveness) of components of the host response to the presence of subgingival plaque can place individuals at increased risk of periodontitis. For example, hypo-responsive polymorphonuclear leukocytes (PMNL) are associated with increased risk for periodontal disease in the inherited condition, Papillon-Lefèvre syndrome (PLS). At the other end of the spectrum, hyper-responsive defence cells (either constitutively or functionally hyper-responsive) may cause excessive tissue damage. Such cells (e.g. PMNLs, macrophages) migrate into the periodontal tissues and secrete excessive levels of destructive enzymes and mediators as part of the inflammatory host response against plaque bacteria, resulting in breakdown of surrounding periodontal hard and soft tissues, in a manner referred to as "collateral damage".

While research has identified an important role for genetic factors in periodontitis, and we may be able to postulate that individuals with rare syndromes such as PLS possess defective PMNLs, in the majority of patients who present clinically with periodontitis we are not yet able to make meaningful statements about their genotype (their "genetic make-up"). Furthermore, we are not in a position to be able to alter a genetic profile so as to reduce the risk of periodontitis. It is, however, important to ask about other family members when examining a patient with periodontitis, particularly young patients with aggressive forms of the disease.

Aggressive periodontitis tends to occur in families, suggesting a genetic basis to the disease. The precise nature of any immune defect that is inherited in families may not be apparent. There may be a defect in PMNL function, for example, that predisposes the patient to periodontitis, but does not manifest as any other clinical sign or symptom, and the patient appears to be medically healthy (other than a diagnosis of periodontitis). A detailed family history, including questions about whether brothers or sisters have periodontal problems, or whether the patient's parents lost their teeth early, are also an important part of the information gathered from patients with all forms of periodontitis. Such data help to inform the diagnosis and provide a "window" on the potential "natural history" of that patient's disease, i.e. how their genetic make-up may be expressed clinically (their "phenotype").

Genetic Susceptibility Testing

A commercial test for genetic status in periodontitis patients has been developed. This is the Periodontal Susceptibility Test (PST), which is performed on a finger-prick blood sample. This tests for what has been called the Periodontitis-Associated Genotype (PAG), the presence of specific polymorphisms in the gene that codes for interleukin-1 (IL-1). A polymorphism is not a mutation in the gene, and polymorphisms exist throughout the human genome. In the case of the PST, single nucleotide polymorphisms (SNPs) are identified, in which there is a single change in the base pair sequence in the DNA molecule at specific points in the gene. Research has suggested that individuals who possess these specific polymorphisms (i.e. are PAG-positive) produce more IL-1 for a given bacterial challenge, and in view of the importance of IL-1 in periodontal pathogenesis, they are therefore more likely to have periodontal disease. Indeed, some studies have suggested that PAG-positive patients who smoke are up to seven times more likely to have severe periodontitis compared to PAG-negative smokers, although other studies have failed to identify such an association.

This raises the question, if a patient is PAG-positive, should they be managed any differently from those who are PAG-negative, either before periodontal disease has developed, during periodontal treatment, or during the supportive phase of periodontal therapy? At the present time, there is simply not enough evidence that patients should be managed any differently on the basis of available genetic tests such as the PST. For example, the association between PAG and periodontitis was only seen in smokers. When non-smokers were included in the analysis, no association was apparent. Furthermore, associations between particular genes and periodontal disease have only been demonstrated in certain populations (typically, white Caucasians), and not in other racial or ethnic groups. It is clear, therefore, that genetic tests based upon specific genes may not apply to all patients. Importantly, studies in the UK and Europe indicate that a test such as PST is of little benefit for these populations, but the future holds exciting possibilities for risk factor identification, early diagnosis, and improved management strategies that have a strong scientific basis. Finally, the associations between genes and disease may be indirect, i.e. the presence of a certain genotype does not directly impact on the disease. Instead, there may be interactions between genetic factors and other risk factors (such as smoking) and, therefore, the genotype may only be relevant if other risk factors are also present.

What do genetic test results mean, and what is their impact on the patient?

In all the studies that have evaluated PAG and periodontal disease, there have been substantial numbers of patients who were PAG-positive who did not have periodontal disease and, conversely, large numbers of patients who were PAG-negative who did have periodontal disease. Clearly, PAG status (as identified by the PST) does not directly impact on periodontal status in all patients. Patient considerations must also be taken into account when performing any genetic test, and patients must be counselled before undergoing such a test. Genetic testing could theoretically have negative effects on individual patients. For example, a PAG-positive patient might think that they will inevitably develop periodontal disease no matter what they do, and they may therefore fail to comply with periodontal preventive strategies or oral hygiene programmes. Conversely, PAG-negative patients might believe that this makes them safe from periodontal disease, and they may also fail to comply with plaque control requirements. However, just as periodontal disease is polymicrobial in nature (not caused by a single pathogen), it is also poly-immune/inflammatory in aetiology. It is therefore likely that it is polygenic rather than monogenic in nature and therefore a single gene polymorphism, like those tested with the PST, is unlikely to explain the disease risk in most patients.

In summary, caution must be employed when interpreting the findings of genetic susceptibility tests for periodontitis. However, research will continue, and associations between genetic status and the presence of other risk factors such as smoking may become apparent. Currently, there is no evidence to suggest that patients should be treated any differently on the basis of genetic testing.

Environmental Risk Factors for Periodontitis

Drugs Associated With Gingival Overgrowth

Phenytoin (anticonvulsant), the calcium channel blockers (e.g. nifedipine, amlodipine) and ciclosporin (an immunosuppressant) are associated with gingival overgrowth (Fig 4-2). The precise mechanism for the overgrowth is not clear, but involves interactions between inflammatory cells in the gingival and periodontal tissues, the drug, and susceptible sub-populations of fibroblasts in the connective tissues. Gingival overgrowth renders oral hygiene more difficult, which may in turn lead to the development of peri-

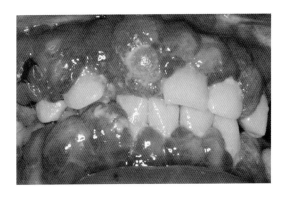

Fig 4-2 Drug-induced gingival overgrowth in a patient taking ciclosporin.

odontitis with attachment and bone loss. Not all patients who are taking these medications develop gingival overgrowth.

The first step in managing this problem is prevention. If the medical history reveals that a patient is taking one of these medications, then they should be informed about the risk of developing gingival overgrowth, provided with appropriate oral hygiene instruction (OHI), and entered into a regular preventive care programme involving reinforcement of OHI and regular prophylaxes to disrupt supra- and subgingival plaque deposits. For the majority of patients, this preventive regimen should be adequate.

In those patients who present with pre-existing gingival overgrowth, clinical examination usually reveals that there is a clear inflammatory component to the overgrown tissues, as a result of plaque accumulation. The first step, therefore, is to provide thorough periodontal non-surgical treatment, including OHI and full mouth root surface instrumentation (RSI) to remove plaque and calculus deposits. Often, in cases of mild overgrowth, this treatment is sufficient to reduce the extent of the overgrown tissues as the inflammation resolves, which facilitates plaque control by the patient. The patient should then be enrolled into a regular supportive programme of OHI and full-mouth prophylaxis.

Liaison with the medical specialist is important in cases of overgrowth that are particularly severe, or recur. It may be possible to switch the patient to a non-calcium channel blocking anti-hypertensive drug prescription. For those patients taking ciclosporin, an alternative that is not associated with overgrowth is Tacrolimus. Gingival overgrowth is one of only two side effects of ciclosporin medication that justification for a change to Tacrolimus (the other is hypertrichosis). Clearly, the decision to switch medication must be made by the medical practitioner or, more often, the medical specialist, after consultation with the dentist.

For very severe cases of overgrowth, gingivectomy surgery may be indicated using either a scalpel or a surgical laser. If surgery is to be performed, it is essential that the patient first undergoes non-surgical periodontal treatment to improve oral hygiene and reduce the inflammatory component of the condition. As the inflammation resolves following efficacious non-surgical treatment, the size of the overgrown tissues is reduced which makes the surgery easier to perform. In the majority of cases requiring gingivectomy, referral to an appropriate specialist centre is appropriate, particularly in severe cases.

HIV Disease
Whilst necrotising periodontal conditions are more likely in HIV-positive patients, HIV status does not appear to impact on the development or progression of chronic periodontitis. HIV-positive individuals with chronic periodontitis should therefore be managed in the same way as HIV-negative patients.

The management of necrotising periodontal conditions is covered in Chapter 6.

Behavioural Risk Factors for Periodontitis

Smoking
Smoking is a major risk factor for periodontitis, and research suggests that over 50% of cases of chronic periodontitis in Western populations may be caused by smoking. Stopping smoking is of benefit to periodontitis patients, with the response to periodontal treatment in former smokers being approximately mid-way between that seen in non-smokers and in current smokers. Dentists have, on the whole, not tended to involve themselves in providing smoking cessation advice. Some of the perceived barriers to providing smoking cessation advice include:
- lack of time in the dental surgery
- lack of training
- patient disinterest
- a belief that other forms of dental advice (e.g. OHI) are more important.

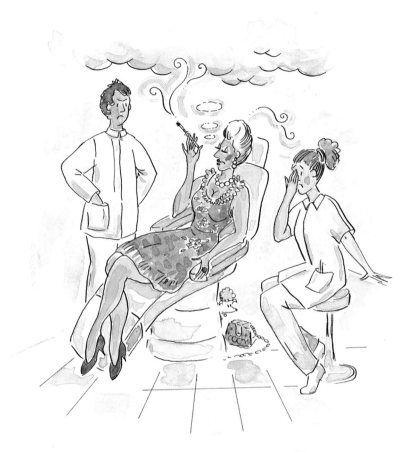

Fig 4-3 "What do you mean, smoking is bad for my gums?"

However, the dental team does have a very important role to play in smoking cessation (Fig 4-3). Most patients visit their dentist every six months, whereas they only tend to see their medical practitioner when they have a medical problem. Furthermore, members of the dental team (particularly dental hygienists) are already trained in modifying patients' behaviour (e.g. in terms of oral hygiene practices), and already possess many of the skills required in helping patients to quit smoking. Helping smokers to quit is a national healthcare priority, and the high number of patient–dental team interactions that occur each year suggests that the dental team is ideally placed as a primary care provider of smoking cessation counselling. As early as 1993, the National Cancer Institute of America recognised that "dentists have a key role to play in providing smoking cessation advice" and research has shown that dentists are as effective as doctors and nurses in helping patients to quit.

At the very least, dentists must record a medical history that includes a smoking history. The number of cigarettes smoked and the number of years for which the patient has been a smoker must be recorded, to enable calculation of the number of pack-years (i.e. the number of packs of twenty cigarettes each day multiplied by the number of years as a smoker). Periodontitis patients who smoke must be informed about the deleterious effects of smoking on the periodontium and this must be recorded in the patient's notes. Patients should also be advised that treatment outcomes are reduced in smokers, although this should not be seen as an excuse to either not provide treatment or to provide substandard care. Patients should also be asked whether they have considered quitting. Discussing these issues with patients is certainly not a waste of time – research has shown that brief advice from a healthcare professional can result in quit rates of 2-5%.

The five key steps (the "5 As") to smoking intervention in the primary care setting are shown in Box 4-1. It does not take long to go through the "5 As", and it is extremely rewarding if a patient quits following intervention. The stages of quitting are illustrated in Fig 4-4. A patient in the "pre-contemplation" stage (a "contented smoker") is not yet ready to think about quitting. The contented smoker will report that they enjoy smoking, and

Box 4-1 **The "Five As" Approach**

Ask *patients about smoking, and record the answer in the notes*

Advise *smokers to quit by providing clear, unambiguous and personalised information*

Assess *whether the patient is willing to make a quit attempt, and, if so, then provide help with this*

Assist *the patient with a quit plan: set a quit date, provide counselling, recommend smoking cessation aids (e.g. nicotine replacement therapy)*

Arrange *a follow up soon after the quit date. Congratulate success. If the patient has lapsed, then consider the circumstances.*

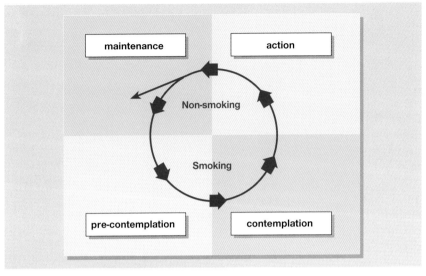

Fig 4-4 The quitting cycle for smokers.

Box 4-2 **The "Five Rs" Approach**

Relevance – *make the importance of quitting relevant to the patient. Motivational information has the greatest impact if relevant to the individual*

Risks – *Explain the risks of not quitting smoking, and try to personalise this information for the patient*

Rewards – *identify rewards of quitting (e.g. improved health, better taste of food, enhanced sense of smell, saving money, better periodontal status)*

Roadblocks – *identify the patient's barriers to quitting (e.g. fear of withdrawal symptoms, fear of failure, weight gain, lack of support)*

Repetition – *Repeat the above each time a contented smoker comes to the dental practice. Most smokers need repeated quit attempts before they succeed* they are not really interested in stopping. For this type of patient, the "5 Rs" are useful to enhance motivation to quit (Box 4-2).

The concerned smoker is one who is in the "contemplation" stage of the quit cycle. This patient is thinking about quitting, and probably has plans to try to quit within the next few months. This is the point in the cycle at which the dental team can be most effective in assisting the patient in their attempt to quit. A quit date should be determined, a quit plan developed, and practical counselling given. External sources of support (e.g. the medical practitioner, or specialist smoking cessation services) can be identified, and a definitive smoking cessation strategy should be formulated.

Smoking cessation strategies are employed in the "action" stage of the cycle at the time of a predetermined quit date. The patient should be aware that total abstinence is essential. All cigarettes should be removed from the patient's environment.

Smoking cessation strategies can be divided into non-pharmacological and pharmacological methods. Non-pharmacological methods include:
• willpower
• advice and counselling from the healthcare professional
• self-help materials
• behavioural therapy
• hypnosis
• acupuncture.

Pharmacological smoking cessation strategies include:
• nicotine replacement therapy (NRT) (e.g. nicotine patches, gum, inhalers)
• buproprion SR (sustained release) (Zyban®).

The success of smoking cessation strategies varies (Box 4-3). Support and pharmacological intervention provide the highest cessation rates. A significant proportion of doctors' practices with appropriately trained staff now run smoking cessation clinics. Liaison with the medical practitioner is essential when assisting a patient in their quit attempt, particularly if the patient decides that they would like to use buproprion, as this can only be prescribed by a medical practitioner. Buproprion was originally marketed as an anti-depressant, but it was noticed that cravings for cigarettes were reduced when taking the drug. Studies have shown that buproprion is very effective in helping patients to quit smoking, and the drug, when properly administered, is safe.

Box 4-3 **Twelve-month abstinence rates for different smoking cessation strategies**

Willpower only	3%
Self-help materials	4%
Brief healthcare professional advice	5%
Brief healthcare professional advice and nicotine replacement therapy	6%
Smokers clinic	10%
Smokers clinic and nicotine replacement therapy	20%

However, interactions with other medications may be significant and for this reason buproprion should only be prescribed by the medical practitioner.

Nicotine addiction is essentially a chronic disease. Most smokers who attempt to quit will cycle through periods of relapse and remission. Different levels of addiction can be treated differently. For example, mildly addicted smokers may require behavioural intervention and NRT only, whereas those with a severe addiction are likely to also need adjunctive pharmacotherapy (buproprion) and intensive behavioural therapy. NRT works by reducing withdrawal symptoms, reducing the smoking urge by sustaining tolerance, and may maintain mood, attentiveness and stress handling. NRT is not a cure for nicotine addiction, but provides nicotine without any harmful smoke. Buproprion works by inhibiting dopamine reuptake and altering noradrenaline activity. It also reduces weight gain. Buproprion should not be used in patients:
• with seizure disorders
• with a previous diagnosis of bulimia or anorexia
• taking other antidepressants
• taking monoamine oxidase inhibitors.

Life-style Risk Factors for Periodontitis

Stress
Stress is a potential risk factor for periodontitis (Fig 4-5). Stress has an adverse effect on immune function, and although the precise role of stress in periodontitis has yet to be elucidated, there appears to be a biological basis for associations reported between periodontal disease and poor coping strate-

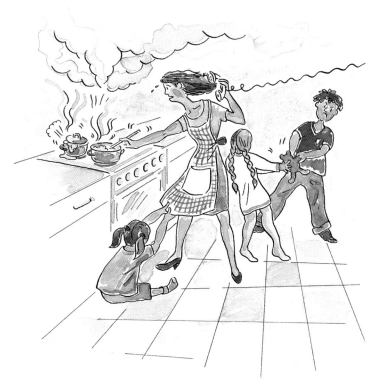

Fig 4-5 "I tell you, if you don't get home soon and help me with these children, I'll get gum disease!"

gies. Stress has long been considered as an important predisposing factor in necrotising ulcerative gingivitis (NUG). Research has also identified that patients with inadequate stress behaviour strategies (defensive coping) are at greater risk for severe chronic periodontitis. Patients with defensive coping are more likely to refuse to accept responsibility for their condition or treatment, adopt defensive attitudes and consider themselves to have better control over situations than others in the same position.

There are two theories as to why psychosocial stress may impact on periodontal disease. The psychoneurogenic model suggests that poor coping with stress results in alterations in neural processes that induce centrally mediated immune suppression and aggravate inflammation, thereby negatively impacting upon chronic inflammatory disease. The behaviour-orientated model considers that stress results in changed behaviour that in turn negatively impacts on health. For example, the patient may be very defensive in attitude, may make light of the disease, may not comply with treatment, and may be anxious (and possibly demonstrate other calming behaviour patterns such as smoking). Poor ability to cope with stress may also lead to neglect of oral hygiene. Furthermore, treatment of periodontal disease is often associated with pain and discomfort and is time consuming and costly – factors that also may be psychological stressors, leading to responses that are deleterious to periodontal health. Recent research has demonstrated that periodontal bacteria are capable of utilising the stress hormones noradrenaline and adrenaline to enhance growth and virulence expression. These reported differential responses might underlie a mechanism whereby the periodontal pathogen can directly take advantage of a "stressed host".

Clearly, the means of managing stress in the dental practice are likely to be limited. The dentist should, however, be careful to ensure that patients receive information in such a way that it does not cause them to become defensive. For patients displaying overt signs of poor coping abilities, liaison with the patient's medical practitioner, with possible referral for stress management therapy may be useful. For those patients who have poor stress management, getting to know themselves through such therapy may be an important part of managing their periodontal disease.

Metabolic Risk Factors for Periodontitis

Diabetes Mellitus

The degree of diabetic control appears to be more important when considering diabetes as a risk factor for periodontitis than the diagnosis of diabetes. Therefore, when treating a patient with diabetes, it is important to ask the patient how well controlled their diabetes is. Most diabetic patients will be aware of whether they are well controlled or poorly controlled. In general, it is best to schedule dental appointments for diabetic patients in the early morning, and they should be told to have their breakfast, insulin injection (if insulin controlled) or medication as normal prior to coming to the surgery. There is no indication to cover routine dental procedures with systemic antibiotics in diabetic patients.

The factors that contribute to increased risk for periodontitis in diabetic patients have already been described in *Understanding Periodontal Diseases: Assessment and Diagnostic Procedure in Practice*. Studies have shown that populations of diabetic patients tend to contain about twice as many patients with advanced periodontitis as do non-diabetic populations. When treating the diabetic patient with periodontitis, it is important to explain the relationship between the two diseases to the patient, and to emphasise in a positive way the importance of complying with OHI, periodontal treatment, and supportive care. Liaison with the medical practitioner is important in poorly controlled diabetic patients to ascertain the reasons for the poor control. There is also some evidence that successful treatment of periodontitis may facilitate diabetic control, and therefore, even in poorly controlled cases, periodontal treatment should be performed meticulously. Finally, it is estimated that nearly half of cases of diabetes are undiagnosed, and therefore in those patients with very aggressive forms of periodontitis it may be prudent to consult with the patient's doctor for appropriate diabetes evaluation.

Other Systemic Risk Factors for Periodontitis

Other systemic risk factors for periodontitis have been described in *Understanding Periodontal Diseases: Assessment and Diagnostic Procedure in Practice*. These include risks such as haematological diseases (e.g. leukaemias, agranulocytosis, neutropenias), disorders such as sarcoidosis, and Crohn's disease, and inherited conditions such as hypophosphatasia and PLS. Many of these conditions are relatively rare, and for many of the more serious diseases, referral to a specialist centre may be indicated. However, many conditions can be managed in the dental practice setting, and for these patients an emphasis on prevention is key, with OHI tailored to the needs of the patient and regular supportive care.

Conclusions of Clinical Importance

- Systemic risk factors such as smoking and poorly controlled diabetes impact negatively on periodontal status and response to treatment.
- It is the dentist's responsibility to identify the presence of risk factors, document them in the case notes, and take appropriate action regarding management.
- Risk factor identification and management should form an integral part of the comprehensive treatment of patients with periodontitis.
- Liaison with the patient's medical practitioner is an essential requirement when managing patients with known risk factors.
- Smoking cessation forms a key component in the management of periodontitis. The dental team is well placed to provide smoking cessation counselling.

- The best smoking cessation strategies involve counselling and the use of pharmacotherapies such as nicotine replacement therapy.
- Commercially available genetic tests for susceptibility to periodontitis should not be used to inform treatment-planning decisions.

Further Reading

Chapple ILC, Gilbert AD. Understanding Periodontal Diseases: Assessment and Diagnostic Procedures in Practice. London: Quintessence, 2002.

LeResche L, Dworkin SF. The role of stress in inflammatory disease, including periodontal disease: review of concepts and current findings. Periodontol 2000 2002;30:91-103.

Roberts A, Matthews JB, Socransky SS, Freestone PPE, Williams PH, Chapple ILC. Stress and the periodontal diseases. Effects of catecholamines on the growth of periodontal bacteria in vitro. Oral Microbiol Immunol 2002;17:296-303.

Salvi GE, Lawrence HP, Offenbacher S, Beck JD. Influence of risk factors on the pathogenesis of periodontitis. Periodontol 2000 1997;14:173-201.

Tomar SL. Dentistry's role in tobacco control. J Am Dent Assoc 2001;132:30S-35S.

Watt RG, Johnson NW, Warnakulasuriya KA. Action on smoking – opportunities for the dental team. Brit Dent J 2000;189:357-360.

Chapter 5
Managing Local Risk Factors

Aim

Clinical examination of patients often reveals the presence of local risk factors for periodontal disease. This chapter aims to provide information on how to manage local risk factors as part of the overall treatment plan.

Outcome

After reading this chapter, the reader should:
- be aware of the more common local risk factors that may impact on periodontal disease progression and provision of treatment
- understand better the impact of trauma from occlusion on the periodontium, and how to manage occlusal trauma
- understand the importance of furcation involvement in multi-rooted teeth
- be better informed on how to manage specific local predisposing factors.

Definitions

The concept of multi-level risk assessment was described in *Understanding Periodontal Diseases: Assessment and Diagnostic Procedures in Practice*. Briefly, risk assessment should be undertaken at the patient level, the mouth level, the tooth level and the periodontal site level. In order to identify local risk factors for periodontal disease, a thorough clinical and radiographic examination should be undertaken (Chapters 7, 8 and 9 of *Understanding Periodontal Diseases*).

Local risk factors can be defined as factors associated with the teeth and supporting tissues that may initiate or predispose to periodontal disease. They are difficult to classify, but can be broadly defined under two major groups:
- anatomical risk factors
- iatrogenic risk factors

However, certain risk factors may fall into both groups, such as trauma from occlusion, which may result, for example, from malaligned or over-erupted teeth (anatomical risk factors) or poorly contoured restorations (iatrogenic risk factors). For the purpose of this chapter, trauma from occlusion will be discussed separately from the two major groups.

Trauma from occlusion

Trauma from occlusion can be divided into two major categories:
- traumatic incisor relationships that result in direct damage to the periodontal tissues
- occlusal trauma arising from occlusal interferences that may affect both healthy (primary occlusal trauma) and periodontally-involved (secondary occlusal trauma) teeth (see *Decision-Making for the Periodontal Team*).

Traumatic Incisor Relationships
A complete overbite onto the gingival soft tissues can result in extensive gingival recession with the soft tissues being sheared away from the root surface during function. The nature of the incisal relationship can be classified (Box 5-1). From the periodontal point of view, the Akerly class II and III incisal relationships are most significant (Figs 5-1 and 5-2). With the stripping of the gingiva, loss of attachment occurs, most frequently in relation to the palatal aspect of maxillary incisors and the labial aspect of the mandibular incisors. Akerly class I and IV incisal relationships typically present with minimal, if any, effect on the periodontal supporting tissues.

Box 5-1 **The Akerly classifications of traumatic incisor relationships**

Class I	*Lower incisors impinge onto the palatal mucosa, posterior to the palatal gingival margins of the maxillary anterior teeth*
Class II	*Lower incisors occlude onto the palatal gingival margins of the maxillary anterior teeth*
Class III	*A deep traumatic overbite (class II division 2 incisal relationship) with shearing of the mandibular labial gingiva*
Class IV	*Lower incisors occlude with the palatal surfaces of the upper incisors, leading to tooth wear by attrition*

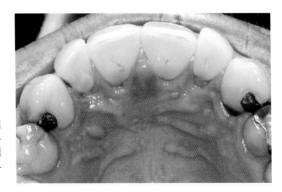

Fig 5-1 Akerly Class II incisal relationship. Note the recession in relation to the palatal aspects of the maxillary incisors.

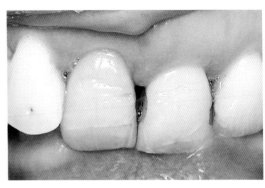

Fig 5-2 Traumatic overbite (Akerly Class III incisal relationship). Notice how the maxillary incisors are impinging on the labial gingiva of the lower incisors (see also Fig 5-3).

Predisposing factors for traumatic relationships include:
- a severe class II, division two incisor relationship
- loss of posterior support, particularly if associated with over-closure of the remaining anterior teeth
- poorly designed anterior restorations with no occlusal stops, leading to over-eruption of the incisors
- incomplete orthodontic treatment.

Frequently, deep localised recession defects will develop which are difficult to keep clean, leading to significant accumulation of plaque and the development of gingival inflammation and periodontal breakdown (Fig 5-3). The first line of treatment is to re-establish gingival health by undertaking non-surgical periodontal therapy and by providing intensive oral hygiene instruction (OHI). Single-tufted brushes may be particularly useful to clean into the recession defect. A useful preliminary treatment option is to provide a

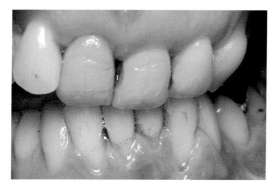

Fig 5-3 When the patient opens their mouth, the consequences of the traumatic overbite can be seen. There is localised gingival recession affecting the mandibular incisors and shearing away of the gingiva, in particular, in relation to the lower left lateral incisor. There is also evidence of attritive toothwear affecting the left lateral incisor.

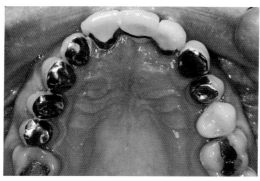

Fig 5-4 Adhesive palatal shims and anterior bridgework to rebuild the anterior dentition and provide a stable occlusion.

soft splint to prevent further damage to the periodontal soft tissues, particularly in those patients with a night time bruxing habit.

Once periodontal health has been re-established, definitive treatment options may be explored. Often, these may be intensive and complicated, and referral for advice and treatment planning by a specialist restorative dentist is likely to be required. Treatment options include:

• Provision of posterior support to re-establish the correct occlusal vertical dimension and eliminate the destructive incisal contacts.
• Restoration of the anterior teeth to provide occlusal stops, e.g. by the provision of adhesive metal palatal shims (Fig 5-4), composite resin restorations, or carefully designed crowns. A "Dahl approach" may be required to increase space anteriorly for the provision of these restorations. The classic Dahl appliance is rarely used nowadays. Palatal composite restorations that have been carefully contoured are equally effective (Fig 5-5).

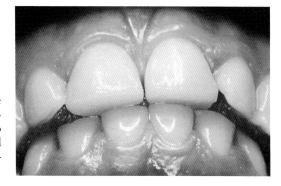

Fig 5-5 Palatal composite restorations used as an alternative to a Dahl appliance to increase the occlusal vertical dimension and provide occlusal stability.

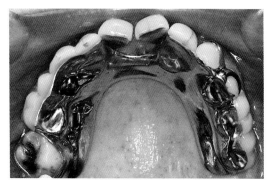

Fig 5-6 Overlay partial denture to prevent further trauma from occlusion and provide occlusal stability.

- Overlay appliances may be used as a long-term alternative to the soft splint (Fig 5-6).
- More complex cases may require orthodontic therapy, orthognathic surgery, or segmental or full-mouth rehabilitation.

Occlusal Interferences

Occlusal interferences and premature contacts can arise when the occlusal morphology and position of teeth are altered following the placement of restorations or after orthodontic treatment. Interferences may lead to occlusal trauma that manifests clinically as:
- increasing mobility and migration of the teeth
- pain
- tenderness to percussion
- tooth fracture
- faceting of cusps

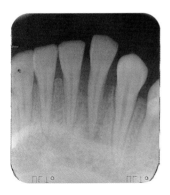

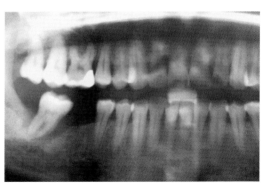

Fig 5-7 Widened periodontal membrane space as a result of a traumatic occlusal interference in a tooth with normal periodontal supporting structures.

Fig 5-8 Crater defect around the lower right molar, which has pre-existing periodontitis and a traumatic occlusal interference (see also Figs 5-9 and 5-10). The bone loss has extended to the apex of the tooth. Notice that there is generalised moderate to severe chronic periodontitis affecting the rest of the dentition.

- bruxism
- temporomandibular dysfunction (TMD).

Occlusal trauma arising from occlusal interferences can be divided into:
- *primary occlusal trauma* in which a lesion results from application of excessive occlusal forces to a tooth with normal periodontal supporting structures (Fig 5-7).
- *secondary occlusal trauma* in which the lesion affects the periodontium of a tooth with reduced periodontal support because of current periodontal disease (Figs 5-8 to 5-10). The greater the amount of periodontal support that has been lost, the more significant the role of occlusion becomes as a co-destructive factor.

The designation of "primary" or "secondary" occlusal trauma is principally for diagnostic purposes. The changes that occur in the periodontium as a result of trauma from occlusion are the same whether there is normal or reduced periodontal support. The diagnosis is often confirmed radiographically. Primary occlusal trauma results in a widened periodontal membrane space (PMS) and early "funnelling" but normal alveolar bone height (Fig 5-7), whereas secondary occlusal trauma presents with obvious alveolar bone

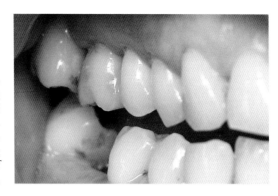

Fig 5-9 Clinical appearance of the traumatic occlusal interference (case illustrated in Fig 5-8). Note the deflective contact between the buccal surface of the lower right molar, and the palatal cusp of the upper right second molar.

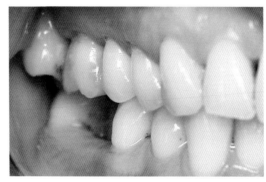

Fig 5-10 As the patient closes fully into the intercuspal position, the lower right molar is deflected lingually. This "jiggling" force affecting a tooth with pre-existing periodontitis has resulted in exacerbation of the destructive events in the periodontium, and is an example of secondary occlusal trauma.

destruction and a characteristic crater-defect surrounding the affected tooth (Fig 5-8).

The lesion of occlusal trauma usually arises following a succession of opposing tension and pressure forces on the periodontium (so-called "jiggling" forces). It is easy to imagine how these arise following placement of a restoration with a high occlusal contact. On the tension side there is increased vascular permeability, collagen and alveolar bone turnover, and on the pressure side there is increased vascular permeability, degeneration of collagen fibres, and bone and cementum resorption. These changes result in a widened, funnel-shaped PMS in which the periodontal fibres have lost their normal functional orientation, and the tooth may become mobile. Over time, significant alveolar bone loss may occur, resulting in a crater-like defect around the tooth.

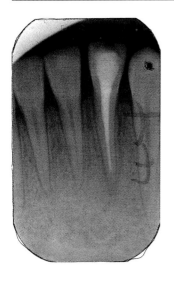

Fig 5-11 Same tooth as Fig 5-7. Following removal of the occlusal interference and root canal therapy, the periodontal membrane space has returned to normal.

There has been much interest in whether or not occlusal trauma can initiate periodontal disease. However, many of the studies that suggested that this might be the case were flawed by using inappropriate animal models and unrealistic occlusal forces. Research has now clearly shown that occlusal trauma does not initiate gingivitis, periodontitis or pocket formation in the absence of plaque-induced inflammation. Also, bone changes occurring as a result of trauma from occlusion without plaque-induced inflammation are reversible once the traumatising forces are eliminated (Fig 5-11).

The changes seen in *primary occlusal trauma* are reversible when the force is eliminated, or the tooth moves out of the influence of the interference and stabilises in a new position. There is no alteration in the connective tissue attachment level to the tooth. In other words, the occlusal interference does not result in periodontal attachment loss. Treatment in this situation will involve:
- identifying the occlusal interference by careful history taking and occlusal examination
- study models mounted in the retruded contact position on a semi-adjustable articulator. Such models are useful to help identify the interference and to plan and assess the likely outcome of removing the interference
- elimination of the occlusal interference by selective grinding.

Following treatment, the lesion should resolve, symptoms subside, and the widened PMS seen radiographically should return to normal.

Secondary occlusal trauma is trauma to a tooth that is already periodontally diseased (Figs 5-8 to 5-10). The occlusal trauma may accelerate the disease process, but cannot initiate disease. Secondary occlusal trauma may increase the intensity or spread of inflammation in already-diseased periodontal tissues, thereby exacerbating the inflammatory host response to the presence of plaque, and leading to increased breakdown of periodontal ligament and alveolar bone. Treatment of secondary occlusal trauma involves:

- careful examination, including identification of traumatic interferences, and full periodontal examination, with radiographs
- treatment of the periodontal condition as a priority. This will involve OHI and thorough root-surface instrumentation (RSI) to re-establish periodontal health
- identification and elimination of the deflective occlusal interference (see above).

Treatment of the periodontal condition should be a priority because, regardless of the traumatic forces present, the regeneration of alveolar bone will not occur following elimination of the interference if plaque-induced periodontal inflammation is still present.

When examining a patient with mobile teeth, it is important to remember that mobility does not necessarily indicate trauma from occlusion. Mobility results from alveolar bone loss (e.g. following previous periodontal breakdown) and may simply be the physiological response of a healthy, albeit reduced, periodontium to normal function. A diagnosis of trauma from occlusion requires evidence of active injury.

Anatomical Risk Factors

Furcation Involvement

Furcation lesions arise when attachment loss occurs vertically and horizontally between the roots of multi-rooted teeth. Furcations are detected during the clinical examination using a furcation probe (Fig 5-12) and by radiographic examination (Fig 5-13). It is important to remember that furcation lesions that are evident clinically may not be evident radiographically, and vice versa. The classification system in Box 5-2 is used to grade the severity of the furcation involvement.

Clearly, for furcation involvement to occur, there must be pre-existing periodontitis that has resulted in attachment and bone destruction down to the level at which the roots divide. Once the furcation is involved in the disease process, treatment becomes much more complicated because it is very difficult for the clinician to gain access into the furcation and for the patient to maintain effective oral hygiene in this area. Reasons include:

- The furcation entrance is often narrower than the tip of a curette or an

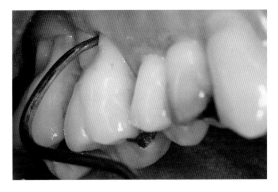

Fig 5-12 Curved furcation probe used to detect a furcation lesion.

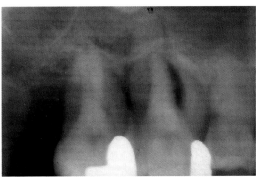

Fig 5-13 Radiographic appearance of a furcation lesion with evidence of interradicular bone loss. This appearance reflects the pattern of attachment loss and bone resorption in both horizontal and vertical directions.

Box 5-2 **Classification system for furcation involvement**

Class I	*Horizontal attachment loss less than one-third the buccolingual width of the tooth*
Class II	*Horizontal attachment loss greater than one-third the buccolingual width of the tooth, but not complete horizontal attachment loss*
Class III	*Complete horizontal attachment loss "through-and-through" destruction of the periodontal tissues in the furcation*

ultrasonic tip, thereby preventing instrumentation inside the furcation (Fig 5-14).

- The furcal surfaces of the roots of multi-rooted teeth tend to be concave (Fig 5-14), creating plaque retentive areas that are extremely difficult to access for instrumentation.
- The roof of the furcation is located more coronally than the entrances to the furcation, further compounding the difficulties of undertaking RSI.

Treatment options for furcation-involved teeth are dependent on the severity of the furcation lesion. The focus must be on effective plaque control, and time must be spent educating the patient in the use of single-tufted and bottle brushes to clean the furcation effectively. Non-surgical treatment options for furcations include OHI and RSI, which may be the only treatment necessary providing that healing results in furcation morphology that is optimal for patient-performed plaque control. Non-surgical treatment is likely to be most successful in class I and, to a lesser extent, class II furcation lesions.

More complex surgical treatment approaches may be appropriate for class II and class III furcations, and frequently a referral to a specialist periodontist will be indicated. Given the technical difficulty of undertaking many of the surgical treatment options, most of which are very technique-sensitive, it is not recommended to perform these procedures without appropriate training. Detailed description of the various surgical options for furcations, together with an assessment of their advantages and disadvantages, is not within the scope of this book. Briefly, however, surgical treatment for furcation lesions may include:

- RSI undertaken in conjunction with flap surgery to improve access
- furcationplasty to alter the furcation morphology to create better access for plaque control and maintenance
- tunnel preparation to convert a class II furcation in a mandibular molar into a class III furcation, which is easier to clean with bottle brushes
- guided tissue regeneration (GTR) and guided bone regeneration (GBR) to regenerate lost attachment
- root resection and tooth hemisection in which severely periodontally-involved roots are removed.

It should also be remembered that the prognosis for furcation-involved teeth tends to be poor. Therefore, extraction of the tooth must always remain an option.

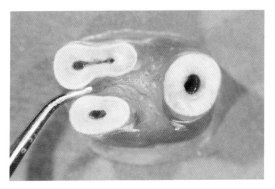

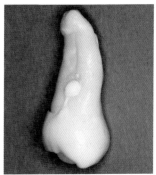

Fig 5-14 The entrance to the buccal furcation in this maxillary first molar is too narrow to permit access for adequate instrumentation. Note also the concave furcal (inner) aspect of the mesiobuccal root, creating a plaque stagnation area.

Fig 5-15 Enamel pearl on the root surface of a two-rooted (fused roots) extracted premolar. Note the cervical enamel projection extending from the cementoenamel junction to the enamel pearl forming a "bridge" of enamel along the root surface.

Enamel Pearls

Enamel pearls are uncommon "droplets" of enamel found on the root surface (Fig 5-15). They may be isolated or linked to the cemento-enamel junction (CEJ) by a ridge of enamel. They have no connective tissue attachment. If present within a periodontal pocket, enamel pearls may be mistaken for calculus, and make effective RSI difficult. If identified, enamel pearls can be removed using a diamond bur, although care must be exercised as, occasionally, larger enamel pearls may contain dentine and possibly even pulp tissue.

Cervical Enamel Projections

Cervical enamel projections (CEPs) are projections of the CEJ into the furcation region of multi-rooted teeth (Fig 5-15). The periodontal attachment to the enamel of a CEP is epithelial, which may make these sites more susceptible to periodontal disease progression. There is evidence that isolated furcation involvements occurring in patients who are otherwise periodontally healthy may be associated with the presence of CEPs. Where access permits, the CEP should be removed because connective tissue will not attach to enamel. This, however, is a procedure that is usually only possible during periodontal surgery.

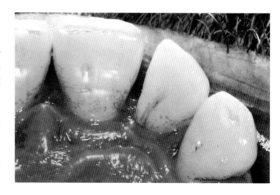

Fig 5-16 Palatoradicular groove associated with deep pocketing on the palatal aspect of this upper lateral incisor. Such grooves may extend close to the apex of the tooth and are, therefore, often impossible to treat successfully by non-surgical management alone.

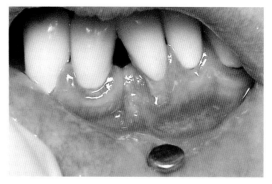

Fig 5-17 Localised gingival recession affecting the lower left central incisor associated with a lip stud.

Root Morphology

Root grooves are plaque retentive features that may be associated with localised, deep, narrow periodontal pockets that do not respond to RSI. Palatoradicular grooves are frequently found at the palatal aspects of maxillary lateral incisors (Fig 5-16), and may extend as far as the apical third of the root. It is impossible to completely remove plaque and calculus from these grooves using a conventional approach, and it may be necessary to raise a surgical flap and perform careful odontoplasty to eliminate the groove. In deeper grooves, there may be communications with the pulp system of the tooth, and in such cases odontoplasty must be undertaken with extreme care.

Gingival Recession

Localised gingival recession is associated with factors such as:
- toothbrush trauma
- high frenal attachment
- habits or factitious (self-inflicted) injury

73

- body piercing (Fig 5-17)
- bony dehiscences, or thin alveolar bone.

Generalised gingival recession occurs in progressing periodontal disease, or following resolution of inflammation as a result of periodontal treatment.

Localised gingival recession results in a reduction in the width of keratinised gingiva. It is important to remember that absence of keratinised gingiva does not inevitably lead to gingival recession, providing a high standard of plaque control is maintained. Localised gingival recession results in exposure of the root surface, which may be aesthetically unacceptable, and lead to hypersensitivity, and an increased risk of root caries.

Treatment options for gingival recession include:
- Recording the extent of the recession by clinical probing and measurement, photographs and study models.
- Eliminating aetiological factors such as a traumatic toothbrushing technique.
- The use of single-tufted brushes to clean into the recession defect.
- RSI to remove plaque and calculus.
- a gingival veneer to cover exposed roots and embrasure spaces, if aesthetics are a concern.

If these treatment options are not successful, then mucogingival surgery may be indicated to increase the width of the attached gingiva or to undertake a grafting procedure, possibly in combination with a coronal advancement flap to cover the area of recession. Referral to a specialist periodontist is likely to be required.

Furcation Ridges
Furcation ridges are pronounced ridges of cementum that run across the roof of a furcation. Furcation ridges, in addition to the concavities of the furcal aspects of the roots, create plaque-retentive areas that are extremely difficult to instrument. Where accessible, they can be removed using small diamond burs (odontoplasty).

Dental Anatomy and Tooth Arch Relationships
The shape of the teeth and the location of teeth within the arch may result in plaque-retentive areas, for example:
- crowding, in which overlapping teeth create stagnation areas in the absence of effective OHI (Fig 5-18)

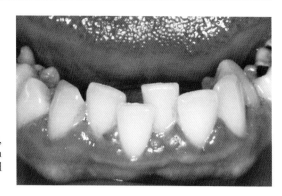

Fig 5-18 Instanding incisors, resulting in plaque stagnation areas and resultant gingival inflammation.

- tight contacts, which make interproximal cleaning with floss impossible
- tipped or drifted teeth, mesially inclined molars, for example, following loss of the mesial neighbouring tooth, resulting in plaque stagnation areas
- bulbous clinical crowns, which predispose to the accumulation of plaque below the line of maximum contour
- prominent cervical features that are plaque stagnation areas
- stacked molars restricting access for cleaning. In such situations the thin plates of interproximal bone are susceptible to rapid resorption if disease develops.

Treatment options for these various situations are very limited, and primarily involve identifying the problem, making the patient aware of it, and providing pertinent OHI to maximise plaque control in such stagnation areas.

Iatrogenic Risk Factors

Overhanging Restorations
These result from poor restorative technique, in particular in relation to gingival margins. Interproximal cleaning is impossible if overhangs are present, resulting in plaque stagnation areas. This predisposes the site to plaque-induced inflammation, loss of attachment and alveolar bone destruction (Fig 5-19). Secondary caries is also likely to develop.

Clearly, prevention is the best option, although even with careful placement and contouring of matrix bands, overhangs do sometimes occur. Treatment options for overhangs include:

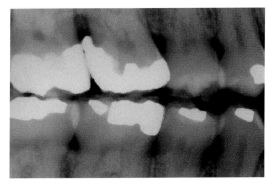

Fig 5-19 Overhanging amalgam restorations and resultant alveolar bone loss. Removal of the overhangs using burs may expose "porous", poorly condensed amalgam on the surface of the restoration. Replacement of the restoration is usually the best treatment option.

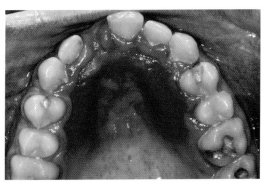

Fig 5-20 Gingival inflammation associated with interproximal collets forming part of a poorly designed, acrylic, mucosa-borne partial denture. The patient also has denture-induced candidosis.

- removal of the overhang (if access permits) with a fine diamond bur, or the use of a safe-sided cutting tip in a reciprocating handpiece
- replacement of the restoration
- following removal of an overhang, OHI and RSI is generally required to remove calculus and control plaque accumulation.

Poorly Designed Partial Dentures

Partial dentures encourage plaque accumulation in the absence of effective oral hygiene. In particular, interproximal collets on acrylic dentures result in plaque accumulation, gingival recession, and breakdown of periodontal tissues (Fig 5-20). Components of cobalt-chrome dentures may also cause direct trauma to the periodontium and if positioned too close to the gingival margins, can encourage plaque accumulation.

Prevention of problems with removable partial dentures is achieved by careful design to:

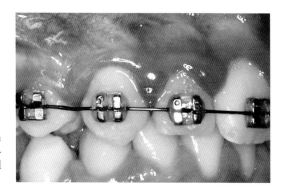

Fig 5-21 Plaque stagnation area and gingival inflammation associated with a fixed orthodontic appliance.

- utilise tooth support rather than mucosal support, where possible
- avoid interproximal acrylic collets
- ensure adequate clearance between the gingival tissues and components of partial dentures.

Treatment of periodontal problems associated with poorly designed partial dentures involves replacing the defective denture with one that is well designed, and OHI and RSI to eliminate periodontal inflammation. Instruction to leave dentures out at night and appropriate cleaning information must also be given.

Orthodontic Appliances

Both fixed and removable orthodontic appliances encourage plaque accumulation. Fixed appliances, in particular, present considerable oral hygiene challenges to the patient (Fig 5-21). Clearly, orthodontic appliances should not be given to patients with sub-optimal plaque control. Appliances should also be designed to ensure adequate clearance of the gingival tissues, with an emphasis on a simple design. Patients should be given intensive OHI, with instruction in the use of orthodontic toothbrushes, single tufted brushes, bottle brushes and floss.

Defective Crown Margins

Defective margins result in localised gingival inflammation. The tissues become very inflamed and readily bleed on probing (Fig 5-22). The most common reason for positive crown margins is unclear margins in impressions, making it impossible for the technician to construct a crown that conforms with the margins that have been created. Treatment options are very

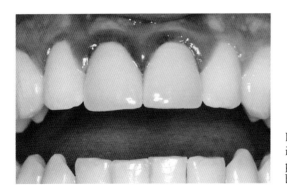

Fig 5-22 Marked gingival inflammation associated with positive crown margins at both central incisors.

limited for defective crown margins. Very slight positive margins may be corrected with a fine diamond bur and careful finishing. Otherwise, replacement of the crown is indicated.

Where possible, crown margins should be located supragingivally so that the gingival tissues are not affected by the crown-tooth interface. If aesthetic concerns prevent this, then crown margins placed at the gingival margin are better than subgingival crown margins as they are easier to monitor and keep clean. Attention to detail is essential when fitting and cementing crowns to ensure the best possible marginal adaptation. Paradoxically, attempts to place crown margins subgingivally for aesthetic reasons usually result in compromised aesthetics because of the development of gingival inflammation associated with plaque retention at the margins. Furthermore, a minimum distance (the "biologic width") of approximately 2-3mm must remain between the crown margin and the alveolar crest. This distance is derived from the dimensions of the dentogingival junction in health, where there is approximately 1mm of epithelial attachment (the junctional epithelium) and approximately 1-2mm of connective tissue attachment. If the biologic width is encroached by placing crown margins too far subgingivally, then inflammation and breakdown of periodontal attachment apparatus ensues until the biologic width is re-established.

Defective Bridge Pontics
Bridge pontics that impinge on the gingival soft tissues result in plaque accumulation and inflammation. This can be prevented by ensuring that pontics are carefully designed to be clear of the tissues and to facilitate cleaning. Pontics should be convex in all directions and have smooth surfaces. A compromise between aesthetics and the ability to keep the pontics plaque-free

is usually achieved by creating minimal, light contact between the pontic and the buccal surface of the edentulous ridge, thereby allowing for self-performed cleaning with superfloss. Treatment options for defective pontics include special cleaning techniques with, for example, superfloss and, where access permits, recontouring of the pontic. However, replacement of the bridge is generally required.

Conclusions of Clinical Importance

- Occlusal trauma affecting periodontally healthy teeth may result in increased tooth mobility and widening of the periodontal membrane space, but does not initiate periodontitis.
- Occlusal trauma affecting periodontally diseased teeth may result in exacerbation of pre-existing periodontitis.
- Vigilance should be exercised when examining patients with periodontitis in order to detect furcation involvement in multi-rooted teeth. Remember that furcations may be evident clinically, but not radiographically, and vice versa.
- Thorough examination of all patients is essential to identify local risk factors and plaque stagnation areas.
- Fixed and removable prostheses and orthodontic appliances must be designed and fitted with great care to avoid direct trauma to the gingival tissues and the creation of plaque retentive features.

Further Reading

Akerly WB. Prosthodontic treatment of traumatic overlap of the anterior teeth. J Prosthet Dent 1977;38:26-34.

Chapple ILC, Gilbert AD. Understanding Periodontal Diseases: Assessment and Diagnostic Procedures in Practice. London: Quintessence, 2002.

Gargiulo AW, Wentz FM, Orban BJ. Dimensions and relations of the dentogingival junction in humans. J Periodontol 1961;32:261-267.

Gher ME. Changing concepts – the effects of occlusion on periodontitis. Dent Clin N Am 1998;42:285-297.

Newell DH. The diagnosis and treatment of molar furcation invasions. Dent Clin N Am 1998;42:301-337.

Noble S, Kellett M, Chapple ILC. Decision-Making for the Periodontal Team. London: Quintessence, 2003.

Chapter 6
Adjunctive Treatments

Aim

This chapter aims to provide a contemporary review of both systemic and locally delivered medications that have been reported for use as adjunctive treatments in the management of periodontitis.

Outcome

Having read this chapter, the reader should be aware of the systemic and locally delivered adjunctive treatments that are available for the management of periodontitis, and should be better able to make informed decisions about the application of adjunctive treatments.

Definitions

"Adjunctive treatments" are those therapeutic interventions that are used in addition to conventional periodontal therapy. They can be divided into "systemic adjuncts", which are systemic medications, and "locally delivered adjuncts", which are delivered directly into the site of periodontal disease activity, via the periodontal pocket.

Systemic Adjunctive Treatments

A variety of systemic medications have been investigated as adjunctive treatments in the management of periodontitis. Systemic medications in periodontal therapy can be divided into two main groups:
- those that are directed against periodontal pathogens (this group includes the antibiotics)
- those that modulate aspects of the host response.

Systemic Antibiotics

Systemic antibiotics are used widely in medicine and dentistry in the management of bacterial infections. Ideally, the decision about which antibiotic to prescribe should be based on culture and sensitivity testing of the infecting organisms, which, in periodontitis, would necessitate analysis of a sub-gingival plaque sample. In the majority of cases, however, this is not practical because reliable and comprehensive systems for analysis of plaque bacteria are simply not available. Furthermore, periodontal infections are polymicrobial involving different bacterial species all with different sensitivities to different antibiotics, which renders decision-making with regard to prescribing antibiotics even more complex. Some of the problems associated with using antibiotics in periodontitis are listed in Box 6-1.

It should be remembered that thorough conventional non-surgical periodontal therapy is effective for the vast majority of periodontitis patients. Therefore, to show an additive therapeutic effect when using adjunctive antibiotics would require research projects with very large numbers of subjects to detect statistically significant results. There has been a dearth of such studies in the periodontal literature.

A further problem relating to antibiotic use is that of bacterial resistance, which can be defined as "a decrease of susceptibility to an antibacterial to the extent that therapy is likely to fail when it is used clinically for a recommended indication". Worldwide, the therapeutic advantages offered by antibiotics are being threatened by the emergence of resistant bacterial strains.

Box 6-1 **Problems with antibiotic usage in periodontitis**

More than 500 bacterial species have been identified in dental plaque, of which approximately 15-20 have been strongly associated with disease.

Most periodontal pathogens are indigenous to the oral cavity, and can be found (albeit in reduced numbers) in periodontally healthy patients.

Periodontal diseases are markedly heterogeneous, and present as a spectrum of change from health to severe disease.

Periodontitis is a clinical diagnosis, not a microbiological diagnosis.

Microbiological sampling systems for culture and sensitivity are not readily available.

There are relatively few randomised studies of the use of antibiotics in periodontitis.

The host response plays a major role in the pathogenesis of periodontitis.

This has primarily occurred because of:
- overuse of antimicrobials
- misuse of antimicrobials
- widespread use of antibiotics in agriculture and animal husbandry
- lapses in infection control
- an increase in the number of immunocompromised individuals.

The solution to this problem involves responsible antibiotic use and stringent infection-control policies. This requires changing the attitudes of health care workers, patients, and the pharmaceutical industry. There is often significant pressure exerted on clinicians by patients who expect a prescription to alleviate their symptoms. If there is no indication for antibiotics, the temptation to prescribe must be resisted and other more appropriate alternatives must be explored. Acute infective episodes are best managed by draining the infection and treating the source of infection rather than by prescription of antibiotics.

Antibiotics and Specific Periodontal Conditions
Chronic Periodontitis
Systemic antibiotics are not indicated in the management of cases of chronic periodontitis. Studies have not established with any certainty whether RSI and systemic antibiotics result in any treatment benefit compared to RSI alone. This is because the microbiota associated with chronic periodontitis is relatively poorly defined, rates of disease progression differ between individuals, and there are difficulties in accurately measuring disease progression and response to treatment. Furthermore, recolonisation of periodontal pockets with periodontal pathogens occurs rapidly following antimicrobial therapy. Given that systemic antibiotics have not been shown to enhance long-term treatment outcomes in chronic periodontitis, they cannot be indicated in this condition.

Aggressive Periodontitis
Following the reclassification of periodontal diseases in 1999 (see *Understanding Periodontal Diseases: Assessment and Diagnostic Procedure in Practice*), the conditions previously termed "juvenile periodontitis" and "rapidly progressive periodontitis" were renamed "aggressive periodontitis". It should be remembered that aggressive periodontitis is rare, affecting approximately 0.5% of the population, and therefore is rarely encountered in day-to-day dental practice.

Localised aggressive periodontitis is frequently associated with *Actinobacillus actinomycetemcomitans (Aa)* infection, an organism that is particularly virulent and possesses the ability to invade the gingival soft tissues. Invasion of the tissues affords the organism a degree of protection from root surface instrumentation (RSI) and allows for rapid recolonisation of the instrumented root surface. For this reason, systemic antibiotics are useful in suppressing this organism. Historically, 250mg tetracycline four times daily for three weeks as an adjunct to full-mouth RSI has been prescribed. Good clinical improvements have been reported, as *Aa* has tended to be particularly sensitive to tetracycline. However, the recent development of tetracycline-resistant strains of *Aa* has led some researchers to switch to an antibiotic regimen of metronidazole (400mg three times daily) and amoxicillin (250mg three times daily) for seven days as an adjunct to full mouth RSI. This combined antibiotic regimen has been shown to result in better clinical outcomes than tetracycline when both were used as adjuncts to RSI in the management of localised aggressive periodontitis.

Generalised aggressive periodontitis is also associated with infection by *Aa*, and also *Porphyromonas gingivalis (Pg)*, another organism that possesses multiple virulence factors and has the ability to invade periodontal tissues. Research studies have reported conflicting data on the benefits of systemic antibiotics as an adjunct to RSI in treating this condition. In patients with aggressive disease, typically presenting with multiple periodontal abscesses, a combined regimen of metronidazole and amoxicillin (as above) can be used as an adjunct to full-mouth RSI. Ideally, full-mouth RSI should be conducted within a short time period (up to seven days) to coincide with the antibiotic therapy. This concept also can be incorporated into one-stage full mouth therapy (see Chapter 1).

Refractory Periodontitis
Refractory periodontitis and recurrent periodontitis (see *Understanding Periodontal Diseases: Assessment and Diagnostic Procedure in Practice*) can be difficult to distinguish. Both tend to result in continued periodontal destruction despite conventional therapy. Given that patients have received appropriate treatment and are enrolled into an adequate supportive periodontal care programme (Chapter 7), refractory periodontitis is most likely to be due to a number of host factors, such as smoking, stress or specific immune defects rather than the presence of a particular microflora. Studies investigating adjunctive antibiotics in the treatment of refractory periodontitis have provided conflicting data. There is no clear answer as to whether adjunctive antibiotics are beneficial, or which antibiotic should be used. This is because of the variable nature of the periodontal microflora amongst patients diagnosed with refractory periodontitis, together with the importance of other

host factors. In summary, therefore, adjunctive systemic antibiotics cannot be justified in this group of patients. Instead, the emphasis must be on excellent plaque control, reinstrumentation to disrupt subgingival biofilms, and risk factor management.

Acute Periodontal Abscess

Patients who present with multiple periodontal abscesses may be treated with adjunctive antibiotics if there is evidence of spreading systemic infection (e.g. raised temperature and cellulitis). The aim of treatment of a periodontal abscess is to achieve drainage of pus, preferably via the periodontal pocket following RSI. If drainage can be achieved in this way, then in the majority of cases the need for systemic antibiotics will be negated. If antibiotics are required, however, amoxicillin 250mg, three times daily for seven days should be sufficient when used as an adjunct to RSI, but the need for systemic antibiotics is the exception rather than the rule.

Necrotising Ulcerative Gingivitis and Periodontitis

Necrotising ulcerative gingivitis (NUG) is an acutely painful condition associated with fuso-spirochaetal infection, smoking, stress, poor diet and possibly HIV infection, characterised by gingival sloughing and blunting of interdental papillae. The condition is so painful that the patient may not be able to brush their teeth. Therapy in the first instance should involve full mouth supragingival ultrasonic instrumentation to reduce the plaque mass, together with chemical plaque control (chlorhexidine mouth rinse) and prescription of metronidazole 400mg three times daily for seven days. Following resolution of the acute symptoms, the patient should be seen for further RSI to remove all tooth deposits together with reinforcement of oral hygiene instruction (OHI). Necrotising ulcerative periodontitis (NUP) may have a similar early presentation although the lesion extends to affect the periodontal attachment apparatus. There may be exposure of alveolar bone, and the lesion is extremely painful. Referral to a specialist centre is appropriate, and treatment will involve local measures, systemic antibiotics, removal of necrotic bone, and possibly periodontal surgery to eliminate bony sequestrae.

Systemic Antibiotics – Summary

The situations in which the use of adjunctive systemic antibiotics may be appropriate are listed in Box 6-2. The key point is that in all cases the use of antibiotics must be an adjunctive therapy. In general, antibiotics are rarely indicated for the management of periodontal diseases, and they are certainly not indicated in cases of chronic periodontitis or gingivitis. The strongest

Box 6-2 **Possible indications for adjunctive antibiotic use in periodontics**

> *Aggressive forms of periodontitis (typically characterised by multiple suppurating pockets) to eliminate reservoirs of bacteria in the tissues.*
>
> *Necrotising periodontal conditions.*
>
> *Periodontal abscess, though the primary goal is drainage of pus, which can normally be achieved by RSI alone, thereby negating the need for antibiotics.*
>
> *Spreading, severe infection with associated symptoms such as pyrexia, gross diffuse swelling, limited mouth opening, difficulty swallowing.*

evidence to support the use of systemic antibiotics in periodontal conditions comes from studies of localised aggressive periodontitis, and, to a lesser extent, generalised aggressive periodontitis, both of which are relatively rare. The objectives of systemic antibiotic therapy (when used) are to reinforce RSI for bacterial elimination and to support the host defence system by killing subgingival pathogens not affected by RSI. Empirical use of antibiotics should be avoided. The plaque biofilm must be mechanically disrupted, as without this, antimicrobials have limited efficacy.

Host Modulatory Therapy

Host modulatory therapy (HMT) is a relatively new concept in the management of periodontitis, and has been driven by improved understanding of periodontal pathogenesis and awareness of the importance of the host response in periodontal disease. The goal of HMT is to enhance traditional periodontal therapies by modifying the destructive aspects of the host response so that periodontal breakdown is reduced and the periodontium is stabilised. Host response modulators are used as adjuncts to conventional periodontal therapy to maximise the treatment response. Careful selection of patients is key when considering any adjunctive therapy. To achieve best results, patients must be interested and well informed about their condition so that compliance is maximised.

HMT represents an emerging area of periodontal therapy. It is very likely that the next ten to twenty years will witness the development of more therapies that modulate different aspects of the host response, particularly in "at-risk" groups such as diabetics or smokers. Various categories of systemic drugs have been evaluated as host response modulators. These include:

- the non-steroidal anti-inflammatory drugs (NSAIDs) (particularly selective COX-2 inhibitors (see below)
- subantimicrobial dose doxycycline (SDD)
- bisphosphonates.

Different HMTs target different aspects of the host response in periodontitis. A schematic to represent periodontal pathogenesis is shown in Fig 6-1, together with target points for HMTs that are currently available and also local delivery adjunctive treatments (discussed below).

Non-Steroidal Anti-Inflammatory Drugs

Non-steroidal anti-inflammatory drugs (NSAIDs) inhibit the formation of prostaglandins by direct inhibition of cyclo-oxygenase (COX). Prostaglandins are key inflammatory mediators in periodontal disease, resulting in inflammation and enhanced alveolar bone destruction. Studies have shown that NSAIDs administered daily for periods of up to three years significantly slowed the rate of alveolar bone loss compared to a placebo. However, the NSAIDs suffer from some serious disadvantages when considered for use as adjunctive treatments for periodontitis. Daily administration for extended periods is necessary for periodontal benefits to become apparent. The NSAIDs are associated with significant unwanted side effects, including gastrointestinal problems, haemorrhage (due to impaired platelet aggregation resulting from inhibition of thromboxane formation), and renal and hepatic impairment. For the future, the adverse effects of long-term NSAID use may be avoided by administration of a selective COX-2 inhibitor. These newer drugs inhibit prostaglandin formation, but do not suffer from the same unwanted effects as NSAIDs. Further research into the use of COX-2 inhibitors as adjuncts to periodontal treatment is warranted.

Subantimicrobial Dose Doxycycline

Subantimicrobial dose doxycycline (SDD) is a 20mg dose of doxycycline (Periostat®) that is recommended by the manufacturer as an adjunct to RSI in the treatment of moderate-severe chronic periodontitis. It is taken twice daily for three months, up to a maximum of nine months of continuous dosing. Early research data claims that at this dose of doxycycline has no detectable antimicrobial efficacy on the oral flora or the bacterial flora in other regions of the body. A 20mg dose appears to exert its therapeutic effect not as an antibiotic, but as a collagenase inhibitor. Collagenases are members of a key group of enzymes known as matrix metalloproteinases (MMPs) that are produced in elevated quantities in patients with periodontitis, and are responsible for a significant proportion of the breakdown of periodontal structures. Early studies, sponsored by the manufacturer, show some benefits for deeper sites in some patients, but further independent studies are needed to identify which patient groups (e.g. diabetics) may benefit more substantially from such adjunctive therapy. RSI must be performed to the very highest standard to achieve the benefits of adjunctive SDD, and the use of adjunctive SDD does not remove this responsibility from the practitioner.

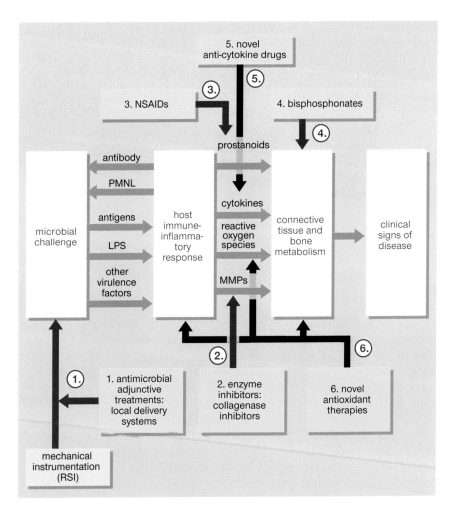

Fig 6-1 Schematic illustration of the pathogenesis of periodontitis and targets/ potential targets for adjunctive therapies (pathogenesis model is after Page and Kornman 1997). The pathogenesis of periodontitis was covered the first book in this series. The potential target points for adjunctive therapies are schematically illustrated. The pink arrows represent possible target points in this pathogenesis model for drug therapies (either topical or systemic) that aim to reduce destructive components of the disease process. The black arrows represent potential therapies, which have yet to be investigated or proven, but which may also form novel adjunctive therapeutic targets. Thus, mechanical instrumentation (RSI) is undertaken to physically disrupt the plaque biofilm: 1.) Antimicrobial local delivery systems may be administered to further reduce the bacterial load. 2.) Enzyme inhibitors (collagenase inhibitors, elastase inhibitors) would inhibit the elevated production of MMPs. 3.) Non-steroidal anti-inflammatory drugs (NSAIDs) may be used to inhibit the release of prostaglandins, thereby in turn reducing alveolar bone resorption. 4.) Bisphosphonates inhibit osteoclastic activity, thereby possibly reducing bone resorption. 5.)/6.) Antioxidant preparations may help restore the balance from excess ROS-production and novel anti-cytokine drugs developed for management of aggressive rheumatoid arthritis may have a role in the future modulation of excessive cytokine activity. The future is likely to see the development of additional adjunctive treatments that target other aspects of the pathogenesis model.

PMNL - polymorphonuclear leukocytes; LPS - lipopolysaccharide; MMPs - matrix metalloprotenases; ROS - reactive oxygen species.

Bisphosphonates

The bisphosphonates are bone-seeking agents that inhibit bone resorption by disrupting osteoclast activity. Their precise mechanism of action is unclear, but research has shown that bisphosphonates interfere with osteoclast metabolism and secretion of lysosomal enzymes. The ability of bisphosphonates to modulate osteoclast activity clearly has potential to be useful in the treatment of periodontitis. Research in this subject is at an early stage, but animal studies have shown that the bisphosphonate alendronate significantly reduces bone resorption in periodontitis. Some bisphosphonates suffer from unwanted effects, such as inhibition of bone calcification and changes in white blood cell counts. Newer generations of these compounds appear to be less toxic and more efficacious. Future research will continue to address the potential utility of bisphosphonates as adjunctive treatments for periodontitis, and this is an emerging area of investigation.

Local delivery adjunctive treatments

Local delivery devices can be used as adjuncts to RSI. Local delivery systems that have been developed to date contain antibiotics and other antimicrobial drugs in a vehicle that is delivered into the periodontal pocket. The potential advantages of local delivery systems include:
- the drug is delivered directly to the site of disease activity
- there is adequate drug concentration at the site of disease, achieving therapeutic concentrations to reduce the levels of pathogenic bacteria
- therapeutic drug levels are maintained over time at the site, without high systemic exposure to the drug
- the therapy is less dependent on patient compliance.

The aim when using local delivery systems is to deliver and maintain effective concentrations of a chemotherapeutic agent at the site of disease for a prolonged period of time. The ability of the agent to remain in the periodontal pocket may be hampered by the outward flow of gingival crevicular fluid (GCF). In an attempt to overcome this problem, there has been a trend in the development of these agents to move away from low-viscosity gel products, which may be washed out by GCF, to products which are inserted as semi-solid chips or as gels that solidify within the periodontal pocket. An ideal local delivery product would:
- be efficacious
- easy to use
- contain a drug reservoir of sufficient volume to maintain therapeutic drug levels over time
- fill the periodontal pocket in three dimensions
- remain dimensionally stable
- be non-toxic/non-irritant
- have no drug interactions or side effects
- cost effective.

Furthermore, local delivery products should be resorbable once their period of maximal efficacy has come to an end, eliminating the need to be removed.

Local delivery systems can be broadly classified as:
- *sustained release devices*, which are designed to provide drug delivery for <24 hours
- *controlled delivery systems*, which have a duration of drug release of >24 hours. There are five systems that have been developed to date, and these systems are summarised in Table 6-1.

Table 6-1 **Comparison of local delivery systems.**

System	Composition	Trade name	Resorbable (time)	Type of device
Tetracycline fibre	25% tetracycline contained within EVA fibres	Actisite®	No	Controlled delivery
Minocycline gel	2% minocycline in lipid gel	Dentomycin®	Yes (1 day)	Sustained release
Metronidazole gel	25% metronidazole gel in a lipid matrix	Elyzol®	Yes (1-3 days)	Sustained release
Chlorhexidine chip	2.5 mg chlorhexidine in hydrolysed gelatin matrix	PerioChip®	Yes (8 days)	Controlled delivery
Doxycycline polymer	10% doxycycline in a flowable polymer vehicle	Atridox®	Yes (7-10 days)	Controlled delivery

Tetracycline Fibres

The tetracycline fibre system comprises ethylene vinyl acetate (EVA) fibres containing 25% tetracycline (Actisite®). The fibre is flexible and is approximately 23cm long with a diameter of 0.5mm. The fibre is packed into the pocket with a plastic instrument so that the fibre is folded back on itself many times to fill the pocket. The fibre can be cut into shorter lengths to facilitate placement, if necessary. The fibre must then be secured within the pocket by sealing the pocket orifice with cyanoacrylate adhesive. The fibre then releases tetracycline at a constant rate into the pocket for 7-14 days. After this time, the fibre must be removed, which is achieved by the use of a curette. When the fibre is removed, is it usually possible to see the root surface as there is a space between the tooth and the gingival wall that was previously occupied by the fibre. Any residual calculus should also be removed at this time.

Tetracycline fibres achieve very high local tetracycline concentrations (1590 μg/ml, compared to 2-8μg/ml if systemic tetracycline is administered), with very low serum tetracycline concentrations (0.4μg/ml compared to 2-8μg/ml with systemic tetracycline). In other words, the local concentration of tetracycline is more than 150 times that achieved by systemic tetracycline, and this provides a bactericidal dose of the drug in the pocket. Furthermore, because the serum concentration is much less than that achieved by systemic tetracycline, fewer side effects are reported.

Clinical studies have shown that tetracycline fibres result in significantly better improvements in probing depths, attachment levels and bleeding on probing when used as an adjunct to RSI. A suppression of the subgingival microflora has also been reported following the use of tetracycline fibres. However, other studies have failed to demonstrate a long-term benefit, particularly when tetracycline fibres were used as adjuncts in the treatment of class II furcation defects.

Tetracycline fibres suffer from some disadvantages:
- the use of cyanoacrylate to seal the fibre into the pocket may potentially result in the development of a localised periodontal abscess
- the fibre is technically challenging to insert, although with experience it becomes easier
- the fibre must be removed.

Minocycline Gel
Minocycline gel is a bioabsorbable sustained delivery system that contains 2% minocycline in a glycerine matrix (Dentomycin®). It is delivered into the periodontal pocket using a syringe and a blunt cannula. Minocycline is a bacteriostatic antibiotic. A relatively small number of clinical studies have been reported using this system. In one study, when minocycline gel was applied four times at weekly intervals in conjunction with RSI, there were significantly better reductions in probing depths compared to RSI alone (although no significant differences were observed in attachment levels or bleeding on probing). A longer-term study, in which RSI and minocycline gel was compared to RSI and gel vehicle only, found that there was no benefit when using adjunctive minocycline gel in pockets >5mm. There are also reports of benefit when using the gel for implant decontamination, but no controlled studies are available to substantiate this. A disadvantage with the minocycline gel system is that the gel is relatively fluid, and tends to be washed from the pocket by GCF flow, therefore necessitating multiple applications. In summary, minocycline gel does not appear to confer clinically significant benefit to patients when used as an adjunct to RSI.

Metronidazole Gel
Metronidazole gel is a bioabsorbable sustained release device that contains 25% metronidazole in a lipid matrix (Elyzol®). It is applied subgingivally

using an applicator comprising a syringe and a blunt cannula, and similar to minocycline gel, it requires several applications. The manufacturers recommend two applications, seven days apart, with each applicator containing sufficient gel for approximately twenty teeth. When the gel is applied into the pocket, it liquefies and flows throughout the pocket, and then undergoes a transformation into a solid phase, which gradually releases metronidazole for approximately 24-36 hours. The concentration of metronidazole in GCF falls exponentially following placement of the drug, and peak plasma concentrations are observed 2-8 hours after application, indicating that some of the drug may be swallowed following loss from the pocket as a result of GCF outflow. After approximately three days, the product bioabsorbs.

Several studies have reported that metronidazole gel used as a monotherapy results in similar clinical improvements to those achieved by RSI. Other studies have compared metronidazole gel and RSI to RSI alone and have identified statistically significant benefits when using metronidazole gel as an adjunct. Microbiological studies have found that the gel has marginal effects on anaerobic bacteria in the periodontal pocket. This is primarily due to the fact that bacterial plaque exists as a biofilm, which, unless mechanically disrupted, is resistant to topically applied antimicrobials.

Chlorhexidine Chip

The chlorhexidine chip is a biodegradable film of hydrolysed gelatin containing 2.5mg chlorhexidine (PerioChip®). The chip is approximately 0.35mm thick, 4mm wide and 5mm long (and therefore cannot be used in pockets <5mm deep). One end of the chip is curved, and should be placed in an apical direction in the pocket. The site to be treated is isolated and dried. The chip is removed from its packaging using tweezers and pushed into the depth of the pocket. A flat plastic instrument can be used to push the chip fully to the base of the pocket. It is important to keep the area dry during chip placement, as contact with moisture renders the chip sticky and flexible, which may make it difficult to place the chip into the pocket. The chip is self-retentive and delivers chlorhexidine to the site at a concentration of 0.125μg/ml for at least seven days, a concentration that has been shown to inhibit 99% of the subgingival microflora. The chip is not associated with staining of teeth or alterations in taste sensation.

Studies have shown that when the chlorhexidine chip is used as an adjunct to RSI, statistically significantly better probing depth reductions and attachment gains were achieved compared to RSI alone. In studies, over twice as many sites treated by the chlorhexidine chip and RSI underwent >2mm probing depth reductions compared to sites that were treated by RSI alone. Following placement of the chip, the patient should be instructed to brush the area carefully but not floss, due to the risk of dislodging the chip. The chip biodegrades after about 7–10 days, eliminating the need to be removed. Research studies have shown that the placement of a chip in pockets ≥5mm in depth every three months provides the most effective treatment strategy. However, such a protocol has significant cost implications for the patient, which should be discussed at the outset of treatment.

Doxycycline Polymer

Doxycycline polymer (Atridox®) is supplied as two components: the active ingredient, doxycycline, and the delivery vehicle, a flowable, controlled-release, bioabsorbable polymer gel. The two syringe contained components must be mixed at the chairside. The mixed product is then placed into one of the syringes, a blunt cannula is attached, and the product is applied into the pocket. The cannula should be introduced to the base of the pocket and then gradually withdrawn as the pocket is filled. As the product is applied into the pocket, it flows to fill and conform to the pocket morphology. Once the pocket is full, the cannula is withdrawn, and the hardening gel can be packed into the pocket with a blunt-ended instrument. Contact with moisture in the pocket causes the gel to solidify to a wax-like substance that is then retained in the pocket for approximately 10 days. Doxycycline is released in high concentrations for 7–10 days.

Initial clinical studies compared doxycycline polymer to RSI, and found that the doxycycline was as effective as RSI in reducing probing depths and promoting attachment gain over nine months. Further studies have investigated the use of doxycycline polymer as an adjunct to RSI, and identified that significantly better probing depth reductions were achieved by RSI and doxycycline polymer compared to RSI alone. Studies have also demonstrated that doxycycline polymer significantly suppresses anaerobic bacteria in periodontal pockets and, whilst recolonisation does occur following treatment, after six months, total bacterial counts were still more than 60% below baseline levels.

Which local delivery product to use, and when?

Interpretation of data from studies of different products is often difficult because of different treatment protocols and different study durations. There have been relatively few studies directly comparing one local delivery system against another. One study compared clinical and microbiological profiles in 47 patients who received RSI and either adjunctive doxycycline polymer, chlorhexidine chip or metronidazole gel. The doxycycline polymer performed the best, with significantly better mean attachment gains than the other two products, and more sites demonstrating attachment gains. All treatments resulted in decreased numbers of periodontal bacteria immediately post-treatment, but at 18 weeks there were no statistically significant differences in microbiological profiles between the groups. In a meta-analysis of studies that investigated adjunctive use of locally delivered antimicrobials by combining data from several comparable studies in order to evaluate outcomes, local delivery antibiotics were found to enhance the treatment outcome.

When deciding whether or not to use a local delivery system, it must be remembered that RSI, when performed to a high standard, is an efficacious treatment in a majority of patients, particularly in cases of mild to moderate chronic periodontitis. Typically, therefore, the first line of treatment will be comprehensive non-surgical management, involving high-quality RSI. For those sites that fail to respond to initial therapy, repeated RSI performed during the supportive phase of periodontal therapy may be enhanced by the use of a local delivery system. When deciding whether to use a local delivery system, there are several factors that must be considered:

- cost-effectiveness, in terms of the cost of the product, the number of sites that can be treated with the product, and the likely benefit of using the product
- patient factors, such as compliance with periodontal therapy and oral hygiene regimens
- medical factors, such as allergy or hypersensitivity to components of the product.

In a well-motivated patient who is able to maintain a good level of oral hygiene, the majority of sites are likely to respond well to non-surgical treatment. When some isolated deeper pockets ($\geq$5mm) remain, the decision may be taken to re-instrument those sites to disrupt reforming subgingival plaque, and an adjunctive local delivery device may be used. Conversely, in those patients who are not complying with periodontal treatment protocols and who have poor plaque control, the use of adjuncts is unlikely to be of benefit.

Having made a decision to use a local delivery system, it would seem appropriate to choose a controlled release device that achieves therapeutic concentrations in the pocket over a prolonged period of time, as opposed to a sustained release device that provides drug delivery for only a few hours. The next consideration is the number of sites that need treating. The chlorhexidine chip will only treat one site, and therefore is likely to be the most cost

Box 6-3 **Suggested clinical situations in which adjunctive use of local delivery systems may be considered**

- *Localised recurrent pockets in a patient in supportive phase of periodontal care.*
- *Non-responding sites following non-surgical periodontal therapy.*
- *Peri-implantitis.*
- *Localised suppurating pockets.*

effective option if only one or two sites require the placement of a local adjunct. If there are multiple sites that may benefit from adjunctive therapy, then one of the gel formulations, such as the doxycycline polymer, is likely to be more cost effective. Situations in which the dentist may consider the use of a local delivery system are listed in Box 6-3.

Adverse reactions and local drug delivery

The advantage of local delivery is that systemic exposure to the drug is low, thereby reducing the likelihood of adverse events, whereas local concentrations are high, achieving therapeutic levels at the site of disease. However, the decision to use a local drug delivery system requires the same prudence and care of selection as the use of a systemic drug. Local delivery systems should not be used in patients with a known history of hypersensitivity or allergy to components of the delivery system. Furthermore, there is the potential for development of antibiotic resistance associated with the use of locally delivered antibiotics, although few studies have addressed this issue. Data available suggest that any increase in the proportions of resistant strains immediately after local delivery returns to baseline levels within approximately three to six months. Other unwanted effects such as pain on placement, tooth sensitivity, development of abscesses, or taste alterations all appear to be minimal after local drug delivery.

Monotherapy or adjunctive use of local delivery systems?

Some of the products detailed above have been studied for use as stand-alone monotherapies and have been compared to RSI alone in clinical trials. In those studies in which the local delivery system was used as a monotherapy, the clinical benefits achieved were no greater than those achieved with RSI, which is the current "gold standard" of care for the treatment of periodon-

Box 6-4 **Key points when considering the use of local delivery systems**

- The therapy must be used as an adjunct to root surface instrumentation.
- The use of a local delivery adjunct does not lessen the requirement for thorough root surface instrumentation to be performed to the highest standard.
- The local delivery adjunct must not be substituted for meticulous oral hygiene by the patient and thorough oral hygiene instruction by the clinician.
- The greatest potential for successful outcomes with local delivery systems may be to enhance therapy at localised, persistent sites that failed to respond to initial therapy in well-motivated patients with good oral hygiene.
- Locally delivered antimicrobials are not indicated routinely where efficacious results can be achieved by high quality, thorough root surface instrumentation.

titis. Using a local delivery system as a monotherapy is likely to be ineffective because of the inability of the therapy to disrupt the plaque biofilm, and the failure to remove calculus.

Therefore, it is essential that locally delivered treatments are used as adjuncts to RSI. Dental plaque exists as a biofilm, which serves to protect individual bacteria within the plaque mass, and therefore such bacteria become relatively resistant to killing by antimicrobial agents. For this reason, the biofilm must be mechanically disrupted by RSI during periodontal therapy. This is true for both initial periodontal therapy, and long-term periodontal supportive care. If subgingival plaque is regularly disrupted by RSI, then conditions favourable for periodontal healing are promoted. Key points when considering the use of adjunctive local delivery systems are shown in Box 6-4.

Key points of clinical importance

- Conventional periodontal treatment is effective in most cases of periodontitis, providing it is thoroughly performed.
- Adjunctive treatments must be used in the manner suggested by their name – as adjuncts to RSI.
- Systemic antibiotics are rarely indicated in periodontics, and are not indicated in the treatment of chronic periodontitis or gingivitis.

- If systemic antibiotics are used, they should be used as adjuncts to conventional periodontal treatment.
- The possible indications for adjunctive systemic antibiotics are aggressive forms of periodontitis, necrotising periodontal conditions and periodontal abscesses.
- Host modulatory therapies are currently being developed and evaluated with a view to correcting defined abnormalities in the host response to microbial plaque. Future, novel therapies are likely to be developed in this area, rather than the more traditional antimicrobial arena, for the treatment of periodontal diseases.
- Local delivery adjunctive treatments are best confined to those situations in which a well-motivated patient with good oral hygiene has demonstrated a good response to RSI in a majority of sites, but there are some persistent deeper pockets that have failed to respond to therapy.
- A variety of local delivery products are available, and the decision concerning which one to use will be determined by factors such as cost-effectiveness, and the practitioner's skill and experience with the product.
- Controlled release devices that maintain therapeutic concentrations in the pocket for extended periods are preferred. These tend to be the products that are semi-solid at time of placement, or solidify in the pocket, to resist being washed out by GCF.

Further Reading

American Academy of Periodontology Position Paper. The role of controlled drug delivery for periodontitis. J Periodontol 2000;71:125-140.

Chapple ILC, Gilbert AD. Understanding Periodontal Diseases: Assessment and Diagnostic Procedures in Practice. London: Quintessence, 2002.

Ciancio SG. Systemic medications: clinical significance in periodontics. J Clin Periodontol 2002;29 (Suppl 2):17-21.

Killoy WJ, Polson AM. Controlled local delivery of antimicrobials in the treatment of periodontitis. Dent Clin North Am 1998;42:263-283.

Killoy WJ. The clinical significance of local chemotherapies. J Clin Periodontol 2002;29 (Suppl 2):22-29.

Page RC, Kornman KS. The pathogenesis of human periodontitis: an introduction. Periodontol 2000 1997;14:9-11.

Walker C, Karpinia K. Rationale for use of antibiotics in periodontics. J Periodontol 2002;73:1188-1196.

Chapter 7

Supportive Periodontal Care

Aims

To provide a comprehensive overview of those aspects of supportive periodontal care (SPC) that follow successful non-surgical management and which are essential to long-term periodontal stability and health.

Outcome

After studying this chapter, the reader should:
• understand what is meant by supportive periodontal care (formerly called periodontal "maintenance")
• appreciate the goals of SPC and how they might be achieved
• appreciate the need for patient compliance
• understand how poor compliance is identified and improved.

Definitions

SPC can be categorised as either primary or secondary.

Primary SPC is essentially preventive and population-based. The aim is to deliver cost-effective dental healthcare measures through community education programmes to limit the development of gingivitis and, in the longer term, to prevent the progression of gingivitis to periodontitis.

Secondary SPC necessitates intervention and may be palliative or directed at the maintenance of post-treatment stability. The aim of *palliative SPC* is to limit or slow down the rate of progression of disease in those individuals who are unable to achieve adequate levels of plaque control. This may be because of poor motivation and poor compliance, or because the patient is medically compromised and unable to undertake effective toothbrushing on a regular basis. In such cases, the removal of plaque and calculus at regular recall visits might help to increase the longevity of a functional dentition.

The aim of post-treatment SPC is to maintain the successful outcomes of periodontal treatment and to prevent, or minimise the chance of, disease recurrence. Post-treatment SPC should be the natural extension of peri-odontal treatment, but may also involve re-treatment of those sites that have failed to respond. This chapter deals with those aspects of SPC that are rel-evant to maintaining post-treatment stability following non-surgical peri-odontal management.

The Rationale for Supportive Periodontal Care

In the 1970s and 1980s a series of classic, longitudinal studies were carried out to assess the efficacy of SPC in patients with advanced periodontitis and who had received surgical or non-surgical therapy. The results of these stud-ies showed that over periods of up to six years, those patients who were recalled on a regular basis for professional prophylaxis, removal of reformed deposits, reinforcement of toothbrushing and the use of interdental clean-ing aids were able to maintain:
- excellent standards of oral hygiene
- healthy gingival tissues
- shallow, post-treatment periodontal pockets
- unaltered attachment levels
- an intact dentition.

Those patients who were not enrolled in an effective SPC programme demon-strated:
- frank gingivitis
- deepening of pockets
- continued loss of attachment
- tooth loss.

In the 1980s, it became apparent that the progression of periodontitis on a patient level did not conform to a linear pattern with time but appeared to follow a more random pattern in which periods of active disease were inter-spersed with periods of inactivity. If the initial treatment phase is inadequate or if some risk factors are not identified then this pattern of disease progres-sion may persist but it will become evident during SPC and re-treatment can then be arranged.

Fortunately, most patients who comply with a SPC programme will achieve periodontal stability, although this can never be guaranteed. Studies during the 1990s confirmed that a few individuals show continued attachment loss despite the very best efforts of the dental team and regular recall visits for SPC. Affected sites tend to show a more predictable and linear pattern of disease progression and it must also be remembered that, although SPC might be considered palliative for such patients, any disease progression is likely to be much slower with SPC than without.

The Goals of Supportive Periodontal Care

The ultimate goal of attaining a disease-free mouth is commendable but is neither realistic nor practical for many patients. The three therapeutic goals of SPC that were identified in a position paper of the American Academy of Periodontology in 1998 accept that SPC should be directed towards limiting disease progression, identifying those sites that continue to break down and providing additional treatment when indicated. The goals are:
- to prevent or minimise the recurrence and progression of periodontal disease in patients who have been previously treated for gingivitis, periodontitis and peri-implantitis
- to prevent or reduce the incidence of tooth loss by monitoring the dentition and any prosthetic replacements for the natural teeth
- to increase the chance of locating and treating, in a timely manner, other diseases or conditions found within the oral cavity.

Clearly, the first objective is achieved by maintaining optimal supra- and subgingival plaque control together with the regular removal of reformed deposits of calculus. However, any programme of SPC must be designed to meet the needs of the individual patient and will, therefore, almost always require a more wide-ranging consideration of the patient's ongoing dental care.

Components of Supportive Periodontal Care

A visit for SPC may include any or all of the following components:
- medical, dental and social histories
- clinical examination and updating records
- radiographic examination
- communication
- reinforcement of plaque control
- continued support with smoking cessation
- supragingival prophylaxis
- subgingival instrumentation.

Medical, Dental and Social Histories
Histories should be updated regularly to confirm the presence of persistent risk factors and to identify new risk factors for periodontal disease. This might

include recording a change in smoking status, an alteration of glycaemic control in a diabetic patient, or possibly identifying the development of stress.

Clinical Examination and Updating Records
The periodontal examination will provide data that should be compared directly either to the pre-treatment measurements or to clinical measurements made after treatment has been completed:
- a formal assessment of the patient's oral hygiene status
- probing depths
- clinical attachment levels including the extent of gingival recession
- furcation involvement
- presence or absence of bleeding on probing (BoP)
- presence or absence of suppuration on probing
- tooth or implant mobility.

The assessment of plaque control should be made at every visit for SPC as this will help to inform the need for reinforcement of toothbrushing measures. The amount of plaque on the teeth tells us very little, if anything, about the disease status of the patient. Nevertheless, the compliance and motivation of those patients who attend for SPC with gross deposits of supragingival plaque might be questioned.

The remaining measurements should be made according to a predetermined time schedule (e.g. at six and 12 months, and then at 12-month intervals thereafter). There is an argument, however, for not probing those sites, which, on usual inspection, appear to have minimal plaque deposits and only superficial gingival inflammation. Sites heal by the formation of a long junctional epithelium and it is important, particularly during the first few months after treatment, that this structure is allowed to adapt tightly to the root surface rather than being persistently traumatised by repeated periodontal probing.

The recording of probing depths and attachment levels are operator sensitive and may show considerable variation, even for the same operator making measurements using the same periodontal probe but on different occasions. This means that a decision has to be made whether a "deterioration" or "improvement" in probing depth is actually a real change or simply a manifestation of intra-operator variability. If a probe with 1mm gradations is used to record probing depths and attachment levels, it is helpful to set a threshold of 2mm, so that a change of 2mm or more from pre-treatment denotes an actual change, whereas a "change" of only 1mm could possibly be due to operator variability. These "changes" can then be highlighted on the patient's periodontal chart (Fig 7-1).

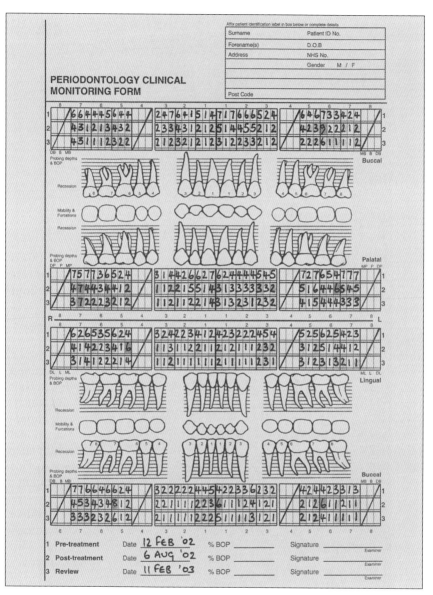

Fig 7-1 Chart showing probing depth measurements pre-treatment and six and 12 months following treatment. If a threshold or cut-off of 2mm is assumed to reflect real change then a useful technique is to highlight those sites that are deteriorating and those that are improving. The deteriorating sites are then selected for retreatment.

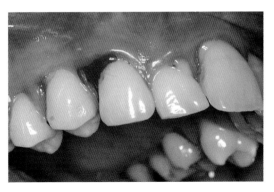

Fig 7-2 Bleeding following gentle probing has traditionally been taken to be a reliable indicator of sites undergoing continued attachment loss. It has now been accepted that bleeding is not a sensitive indicator of disease activity, although, conversely, the absence of bleeding following probing in non-smokers gives a strong indication that the site is periodontally stable.

BoP to the depth of a periodontal pocket has, traditionally, been taken to be an indication of an "active" periodontal site that is undergoing attachment loss (Fig 7-2). Research in the 1990s has determined that only about 30% of those sites that continue to bleed on consecutive visits actually demonstrate additional loss of attachment, thus suggesting that BoP is not a particularly sensitive measure of disease activity. BoP remains a very valuable clinical measurement, however, as an absence of bleeding is a very specific measure of periodontal stability, unless, of course, the patient is a smoker, when such a negative finding may represent a "false negative". Recording BoP can be undertaken at the same time as recording the probing depths.

A complete dental examination may also reveal additional information that is relevant to the ongoing SPC. Dentine sensitivity and, in the longer term, root surface caries may be a consequence of gingival recession and exposure of root surfaces following periodontal treatment. Teeth that were originally deemed to have very poor prognoses might, as originally predicted, become non-functional or develop symptoms to the extent that extractions are indicated. Immediate replacement of the teeth for aesthetic or functional reasons may be indicated and, indeed, may have been planned as a contingency option on the original treatment plan (Fig 7-3).

Radiographic Examination

While radiographs are essential to determine the severity and pattern of bone loss and, therefore, the initial diagnosis of periodontal disease, there may be very little, if any, additional diagnostic yield achieved through repeating radiographs at frequent intervals during a programme of SPC. The need for repeat radiographs tends to be determined largely by the experience and

Fig 7-3 A patient with a history of aggressive periodontitis received an intensive course of non-surgical treatment, although UR1, UL1, UL2 were not saveable. These teeth were extracted and a partial denture provided. During the programme of supportive periodontal care, it was obvious that the patient was able to maintain a high

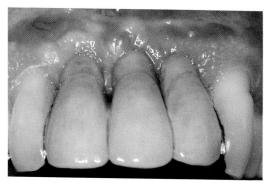

standard of supragingival plaque control, and the prognosis for the abutment teeth to the denture improved significantly. The denture was replaced with a resin-bonded bridge with single abutment teeth.

judgement of the clinician rather than being evidence-based. Nevertheless, it is always useful to have guidelines to follow so that the decision-making process can be applied consistently to all patients:

- In cases where there is little evidence of progressive disease (stable or reducing pocket depths and levels of attachment, and an absence of bleeding on probing), then radiographs might be repeated every two years.
- In cases where the clinical signs suggest disease progression then either intraoral films or a panoramic film might be indicated every 12 months, depending on whether the problem appears to be localised or generalised throughout the mouth. Such signs of disease progression include:
  - deepening probing depths
  - continued loss of attachment
  - increasing tooth mobility
  - continued bleeding on probing and suppuration from pockets
  - recurrent periodontal abscess formation.

Communication

Communication is an essential part of SPC. It is important for patients to be updated regularly on their periodontal condition, areas of persistent disease, the response to treatment, changes in prognosis, the need for SPC and, where indicated, the need for additional periodontal treatment. There must be regular dialogue between all clinicians who are involved in the patient's care so

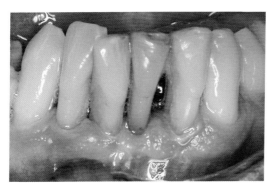

Fig 7-4 A patient with advanced periodontitis who has been in a programme of supportive periodontal care for five years. The standard of supragingival plaque control is excellent. The mandibular incisors demonstrate grade 1 mobility, although the patient is able to function perfectly well and the prognosis for the remaining dentition is good.

that the responsibilities for different aspects of periodontal and dental treatment, together with future management strategies, can be identified.

Reinforcement of Plaque Control

Supragingival plaque control is essential for the establishment of the optimal conditions that are required during the healing stage for 12 months following subgingival instrumentation. Studies have also confirmed that, in the longer term, supragingival plaque control is crucial in preventing or delaying recolonisation of sites with a subgingival flora that is likely to be pathogenic and associated with persistent inflammation and disease progression. That is to say, without adequate oral hygiene, the benefits of periodontal treatment are not likely to be maintained.

The clinician must frequently reinforce the need for effective removal of plaque on a daily basis at SPC visits (Fig 7-4). Those patients who are able to maintain a high standard of plaque removal should be complimented and encouraged. When plaque control appears to be less than adequate, the supragingival deposits should be disclosed, shown to the patient and then the toothbrushing method and the use of interproximal cleaning aids re-evaluated and, if necessary, changed or modified.

Supragingival Prophylaxis and Subgingival Instrumentation

As yet, it is unclear whether supragingival polishing or subgingival instrumentation is the most efficacious and therefore appropriate for the majority of patients in SPC.

A systematic review of six studies that were carried out between 1980 and 2000 concluded that the best available evidence indicates that there is no difference between the two regimes with respect to probing depths and attachment levels at 12 months after the completion of non-surgical periodontal treatment.

The Need for Further Treatment

There are instances when patients, or more often sites within patients, do not respond to an episode of non-surgical treatment. A decision then has to be made regarding whether to consider further treatment as the alternative to continuing with the SPC.

Re-instrumentation of the Roots

There is no benefit of routinely undertaking repeated instrumentation, as this is likely to cause irreversible damage to the root surface and dentine sensitivity. However, even in the most experienced hands, complete removal of subgingival plaque and calculus is difficult to achieve particularly during non-surgical periodontal treatment. Complex root anatomy will compound the difficulty. These sites usually continue to bleed or suppurate because of the persistent inflammation and infection at the base of the pocket. There is continued loss of attachment and the tenacious subgingival calculus deposits can often be detected on the root surface using an explorer. These sites require retreatment and, if access for instrumentation is restricted, then periodontal surgery might be the best option to eliminate the root surface irritants.

The complete removal of calculus from root surfaces might not be essential in those patients who are able to achieve a very high standard of subgingival plaque removal. The consequent resolution of the more superficial gingival inflammation will lead to a reduction in gingival swelling, reduction in pocket depths and exposure of the roots. This will allow more efficient removal of the remaining calculus as an "open" procedure during retreatment.

Adjunctive Antimicrobials

The potential role of locally delivered, slow-release antimicrobials has been discussed in the previous chapter. These agents should only be used adjunctively and following the phases of hygiene therapy and root surface instrumentation. They are not a substitute for inadequate plaque removal, but may be indicated when there remain a small number of sites that appear to be resistant to non-surgical treatment despite adequate plaque control. The sustained levels of antimicrobial drug may be sufficient to eliminate persistent periodontal pathogens at the base of the pocket or situated within the adjacent periodontal connective tissues so that the healing process can begin.

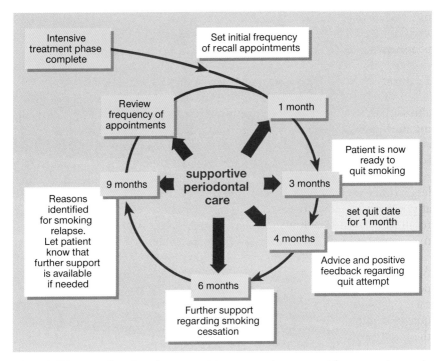

Fig 7-5 Diagram showing the potential opportunity to provide supportive periodontal care and smoking cessation support and advice for a hypothetical patient who suffers from chronic periodontitis that is associated with smoking as a risk factor.

Commencement of the Supportive Periodontal Care Phase

From the practical viewpoint, SPC starts when the instrumentation phase of non-surgical management has been completed. The healing phase occurs within the first two months after treatment. It is during this period that the patient's own plaque control is critical for the successful maturation of the long junctional epithelium. It is important that the post-treatment periodontal probing is not performed within six to eight weeks following the completion of instrumentation because this would disrupt the healing process and would not reveal the full extent of periodontal healing if performed too early.

Further adaptive changes to gingival morphology and consolidation of the connective tissues may occur during the six and nine months following treatment when the position of the gingival margin is likely to stabilise. The SPC should, therefore, be considered crucial to both the healing and stabilisation phases as well as to the long-term maintenance of periodontal health.

Frequency of Visits for Supportive Periodontal Care

The optimal frequency for SPC visits has not been clearly established although there is evidence to suggest that visits for professional tooth cleaning during the initial six-month healing phase should be every two weeks and then on a three-monthly basis thereafter. This three-month interval is based on the approximate time it takes for periodontal pathogens to recolonise pockets following treatment in the absence of SPC. Nevertheless, a three-month recall frequency may be inadequate for all patients; those at greater risk from progressive disease may require a greater frequency of recall whereas those at lower risk and who respond more favourably to treatment may be recalled every six months, or perhaps less frequently.

A schedule that involves more frequent visits in the immediate post-treatment period is logical and evidence-based, but should be integrated with the practical approach of letting the individual needs of each patient determine the frequency of recall for SPC in the longer term. Factors that may directly influence the recall period are given in Table 7-1. Examples of supportive periodontal care programmes for two hypothetical patients are given in Table 7-2.

Managing Risk Factors During Supportive Periodontal Care

Smoking is one of the most significant and prevalent risk factors for periodontal disease and smokers must be made aware of this association. Most smokers have, at some time, made an attempt to quit the habit and many are willing to make further attempts when they learn of the link between smoking and periodontal disease. If a smoker is able to set a quit date that coincides with their periodontal treatment then the programme of SPC provides the ideal opportunity for the dentist or hygienist to provide additional support and encouragement (Fig 7-5).

Unfortunately, when smokers with periodontal disease are successful in quitting the habit they often notice a "rebound gingivitis" and an increase in gingival bleeding as the vasoconstrictive effect of nicotine on the gingival microvasculature is no longer present. Patients should be warned about this possibility and reassured that the bleeding will resolve again once the periodontal treatment has been successfully completed.

Table 7-1 **Factors that should be taken into consideration when evaluating the frequency of recall visits for SPC.**

Less-frequent recall	More-frequent recall
absence of risk factors	smoking, stress, poorly controlled diabetes
good patient compliance	questionable patient compliance
efficient plaque control	difficulty maintaining plaque control
absence of bleeding/suppuration	generalised bleeding and suppuration
shallow pockets	deep pockets
chronic periodontitis	aggressive periodontitis
good response to treatment	poor response to treatment

Compliance with Supportive Periodontal Care
One of the most significant factors that affect the long-term success of periodontal treatment is patient compliance, particularly with SPC. Studies have shown that, even after 30 days, only 50% of subjects are likely to remain compliant with oral hygiene instructions and around 10% will be non-compliant. Furthermore, there are data to suggest that approximately 33% of periodontal patients who have treatment never return for the SPC phase of management and only 15% of patients comply with SPC in the long-term.

There are many reasons for non-compliance with periodontal care:
- a perceived unfavourable treatment benefit
- the time involved
- complexity of the treatment
- cost of the treatment
- stress
- poor relationship with the professionals providing the care
- dissatisfaction with the treatment provided
- the influence of friends and family.

Table 7-2 **Case scenarios of two patients who require supportive periodontal care programmes following non-surgical periodontal treatment.**

Case scenario 1	Programme
A 42-year-old male, non-smoker, with a history of moderately advanced chronic periodontitis. He is very motivated towards periodontal care and is able to maintain an excellent standard of plaque control. There remains one localised 5mm pocket (non-bleeding) in each quadrant.	• Initial recall interval of three months to reinforce interdental cleaning and emphasise the need to clean subgingivally in 5mm pockets. • Undertake supragingival scaling and prophylaxis to remove reformed calculus deposits and plaque. If pockets remain stable and the patient's compliance is maintained then the recall interval may be increased to six months. • Record probing depths at 12 months intervals.

Case scenario 2	Programme
A 50-year-old female with a history of advanced chronic periodontitis. She smokes 25 cigarettes a day, and has done for 30 years. There has been a poor response to treatment. She tries to comply with plaque control, but has difficulties using interdental cleaning aids. Both maxillary second molars are mobile and there are numerous deep pockets (>8mm) that demonstrate bleeding on probing.	• Initial, one-month recall interval to reinforce oral hygiene instructions and to provide supragingival scaling and prophylaxis. • After three months, reevaluate those deep pockets that continue to bleed. Determine need for further treatment as a consequence of incomplete removal of deposits at initial treatment phase. • Tell patient that further advice and support for smoking cessation can be provided if she is ready for a quit attempt. • Lengthen recall interval to three months. If the patient continues to have difficulty with oral health measures, then regular scaling and polishing will become an important part of a palliative supportive care programme.

With periodontal disease, perhaps the principal reason that contributes towards non-compliance is the patient's unwillingness to acknowledge that there is a real problem. The disease is chronic and slowly progressing, only occasionally accompanied by painful symptoms, and is certainly not a life-threatening illness. There is also the belief that it is the responsibility of the dentist, therapist or hygienist to manage the problem. Many patients fail ever to grasp the importance of their own role in the successful outcome of treatment.

Ways to improve patient compliance
Possible methods of improving compliance include:
- Simplify instructions given to patients.
- Remind patients about appointments and ensure that there is excellent communication between the patient and all members of the dental team involved in their care.
- Maintain records of any non-compliance and try to contact the patient at the earliest opportunity when they fail to attend an appointment.
- Inform the patient about the precise cause of periodontal disease. Find out what the patient's expectations are and then discuss the means by which the patient can contribute to achieving these expectations.
- Give positive feedback and constructive criticism whenever possible.
- Try to identify non-compliance as early as possible. Failure to comply with instructions given during the hygiene phase of periodontal treatment will allow the dentist to explain to the patient the likely outcome and reduced prognosis should behavioural change not be forthcoming.

Conclusions of Clinical Importance

- Supportive periodontal care is a crucial component of periodontal management and programmes should be tailored to the needs of individual patients.
- The optimal frequency of visits for SPC should also be tailored to individual patient needs.
- Histories and clinical records must be updated as part of the SPC programme.
- Supragingival prophylaxis is an effective strategy for most patients in SPC but retreatment of pockets that fail to respond may also be necessary.
- Compliance of the patient with SPC is the most significant barrier to the long-term success of periodontal management.

Further Reading

Heasman PA, McCracken GI, Steen N, Sanz M. A systematic review of periodic subgingival debridement compared with supragingival prophylaxis in supportive periodontal care. J Clin Periodontol 2003;30: In Press

Jenkins WMM, Said SH, Radvar M, Kinane DF. Effect of subgingival scaling during supportive therapy. J Clin Periodontol 2000;27:590-596.

Wilson TG. How patient compliance to suggested oral hygiene and maintenance affect periodontal therapy. Dental Clinics N Am 1998;42:389-403.

Index

Index

Quintessentials for General Dental Practitioners Series
in 36 volumes

Editor-in-Chief: Professor Nairn H F Wilson

The Quintessentials for General Dental Practitioners Series covers basic principles and key issues in all aspects of modern dental medicine. Each book can be read as a stand-alone volume or in conjunction with other books in the series.

	Publication date, approximately
Oral Surgery and Oral Medicine, Editor: John G Meechan	
Practical Dental Local Anaesthesia	available
Practical Oral Medicine	Spring 2004
Practical Conscious Sedation	available
Practical Surgical Dentistry	Spring 2004
Imaging, Editor: Keith Horner	
Interpreting Dental Radiographs	available
Panoramic Radiology	Spring 2004
Twenty-first Century Dental Imaging	Autumn 2004
Periodontology, Editor: Iain L C Chapple	
Understanding Periodontal Diseases: Assessment and Diagnostic Procedures in Practice	available
Decision-Making for the Periodontal Team	available
Successful Periodontal Therapy – A Non-Surgical Approach	available
Periodontal Management of Children, Adolescents and Young Adults	available
Periodontal Medicine: A Window on the Body	Autumn 2005
Implantology, Editor: Lloyd J Searson	
Implantology in General Dental Practice	Spring 2004
Managing Orofacial Pain in Practice	Spring 2004

Endodontics, Editor: John M Whitworth

Rational Root Canal Treatment in Practice	available
Managing Endodontic Failure in Practice	Spring 2004
Managing Dental Trauma in Practice	Spring 2004
Preventing Pulpal Injury in Practice	Autumn 2005

Prosthodontics, Editor: P Finbarr Allen

Teeth for Life for Older Adults	available
Complete Dentures – from Planning to Problem Solving	available
Removable Partial Dentures – A Systematic Approach	Spring 2004
Fixed Prosthodontics for the General Dental Practitioner	Autumn 2005
Occlusion: A Theoretical and Team Approach	Autumn 2004

Operative Dentistry, Editor: Paul A Brunton

Decision-Making in Operative Dentistry	available
Applied Dental Materials in Operative Dentistry	Spring 2005
Aesthetic Dentistry	Spring 2004
Indirect Restorations	Autumn 2004
Psychological and Behavioural Management of Adult Dental Patients	Autumn 2004

Paediatric Dentistry/Orthodontics, Editor: Marie Therese Hosey

Child Taming: How to Cope with Children in Dental Practice	available
Paediatric Cariology	Spring 2004
Treatment Planning for the Developing Dentition	Autumn 2004

General Dentistry and Practice Management, Editor: Raj Rattan

The Business of Dentistry	available
Risk Management	Spring 2004
Practice Management for the Dental Team	Autumn 2004
IT in Dentistry: A Working Manual	Autumn 2005
Quality Assurance	Autumn 2004
Dental Practice Design	Spring 2005

Quintessence Publishing Co. Ltd., London